Philosophy and Medicine

Volume 147

The Philosophy and Medicine series is dedicated to publishing monographs and collections of essays that contribute importantly to scholarship in bioethics and the philosophy of medicine. The series addresses the full scope of issues in bioethics and philosophy of medicine, from euthanasia to justice and solidarity in health care, and from the concept of disease to the phenomenology of illness. The Philosophy and Medicine series places the scholarship of bioethics within studies of basic problems in the epistemology, ethics, and metaphysics of medicine. The series seeks to publish the best of philosophical work from around the world and from all philosophical traditions directed to health care and the biomedical sciences. Since its appearance in 1975, the series has created an intellectual and scholarly focal point that frames the field of the philosophy of medicine and bioethics. From its inception, the series has recognized the breadth of philosophical concerns made salient by the biomedical sciences and the health care professions. With over one hundred and twenty five volumes in print, no other series offers as substantial and significant a resource for philosophical scholarship regarding issues raised by medicine and the biomedical sciences.

* * *

Lucien Karhausen

The Fragility of Philosophy of Medicine

Essentialism, Wittgenstein and Family Resemblances

Springer

Lucien Karhausen
DG XII and DG V
European Commission
Brussels, Belgium

ISSN 0376-7418 ISSN 2215-0080 (electronic)
Philosophy and Medicine
ISBN 978-3-031-41632-3 ISBN 978-3-031-41633-0 (eBook)
https://doi.org/10.1007/978-3-031-41633-0

This Springer imprint is published by the registered company Springer Nature Switzerland AG
The registered company address is: Gewerbestrasse 11, 6330 Cham, Switzerland

Paper in this product is recyclable.

To the memory of Micheline Iannuzzelli

Introduction

Arthur Caplan has argued that the philosophy of medicine as a sub-discipline of the philosophy of science does not exist, despite numerous publications and professional activities explicitly conducted in the name of "philosophy of medicine" [1]. He gives the following definition: "Philosophy of medicine is the study of the epistemological, metaphysical and methodological dimensions of medicine; therapeutic and experimental; diagnostic, therapeutic and palliative." Broadbent, in his critique of what he called the "natural turn" in the philosophical literature on health and illness, pointed out the gap between the philosophy of medicine and the great tradition of analytical philosophy [2].

This is the second of my duology on the philosophy of medicine.

In 2023, I wrote a first book entitled Analytic Philosophy of Clinical and Community Medicine, which was the outcome of several decades of research. It offered a coherent approach of the whole domain defined by Arthur Caplan.[1]

The present volume completes the previous one, seeking to identify how my vision of medicine differs from those of the literature: it seeks to illuminate certain methodological aspects of philosophical analysis, particularly in the light of the philosophy of Ludwig Wittgenstein. It also stresses the importance of not straying too far apart from medical clinic as well as from public health.[2]

The philosophy of biology has gained its credentials over the years since the biologist JH. Woodger and Morton Beckner published major works on the philosophy of biology in the 1950s. However, the philosophy of biology became an integral part of the philosophy of science with the publication of David Hull's book [3]. After that, the field expanded and became one of the most exciting new areas of the philosophy of science [4]. The philosophy of social sciences has followed the same trend.

---

[1] *Karhausen L.* Analytic Philosophy of Clinical and Community Medicine. Scientific Philosophy and Philosophical Medicine. Third Edition. 2023.

[2] *Karhausen L.* Les flux de la philosophie des sciences au 20e siècle. 2011.

The philosophy of medicine, on the other hand, has lagged behind. Even though some of the greatest thinkers in the history of philosophy had very important things to say, an important part of medicine has been neglected. Initially, it was mainly concerned with medical ethics, but it has gradually turned its attention to some philosophical issues related to medicine. Often it also consists of a literary reflection on medicine, what Pellegrino calls "medical philosophy", or what Caplan calls "philosophy and medicine", a strategy of a fragmented philosophical approach to medicine, which leads to various speculations as well as to a diversity of contradictory opinions.

In the last 10–15 years, philosophers have begun to understand and work on the conceptual analysis of the problems raised by medical science, medical practice, and public health. In this way, the "philosophy of medicine" has gradually emerged as a vigorous but too often inbred new field, where what is missing is a canon of unified and coherent questions in the context of the philosophy of science [5].

A great deal of work in the "philosophy of medicine" has been done attempting to define such key concepts as health and disease, but it is possible that no definition is ever going to capture all legitimate uses of these terms in the various contexts in which they operate. They may be what Wittgenstein calls "*family resemblance terms*," such that understanding their meaning is a matter of tracking their uses in the range of contexts in which people employ them, understanding their contribution to the forms of life this employment facilitates [6].

This first exercise is based on the philosophy of Ludwig Wittgenstein. Although after the Second World War Wittgenstein considered studying medicine, he did not concern himself much with medicine [7], but his major role in the development of analytic philosophy and his approach to philosophical questions is particularly relevant to this discipline. I found the philosophy of Ludwig Wittgenstein particularly useful in highlighting what separates me from what the philosophy of medicine is today.

The approach of this book is original, as it differs from the current literature on the philosophy of medicine by its bottom-up approach, in contrast to most books and publications on the philosophy of medicine, which use a top-down approach. My starting point is the clinic, public health, and medical research, rather than hypothetical and speculative premises to be defended or rejected.

Although medicine is a profession that has long been linked to irrational and unjustifiable assumptions, it can now be taken for granted that it is both a science and a practice, an *epistemè* and a *technè*; it has epistemic and instrumental dimensions, since it must be seen as a cognitive approach as well as an instrument for producing new techniques for controlling events.

The first chapter provides a general introduction to some recent and significant trends in the philosophy of science.

The second chapter seeks to highlight some of the main lines of Wittgenstein's thought, which are found throughout the rest of the book.

The following chapters deal with the subject matter of medical care in general, including the concepts of physical and mental illness and health.

Next come three chapters covering the separate concepts of causation, explanation, function, and dysfunction.

These are followed by two chapters on the logical and epistemic foundations of medical science and practice, and on teleology, function, and dysfunction.

The question of treatment and prevention is addressed in a chapter that analyses, among other things, the question of placebo and neo-preventive effects and the epistemic difficulties that arise from them.

The next chapter deals with the counterfactual nature of medical explanations.

The last chapter looks at some aspects of the recent development of the philosophy of medicine and the gap between philosophical and conceptual analysis on the one hand, and the reality of the clinic and public health on the other.

Contents

Chapter 1
A Certain Philosophical Context

> Philosophy of science is as useful to scientists as ornithology is to birds.
> *Feynman*

Abstract Moritz Schlick wrote in 1919: "*A philosophy of science does not hope to make the scientific disciplines sufficient and independent, but on the contrary to unify and unite them...Sub specie aeternitatis there is for him only one reality and one science.*"

Keywords Unity and disunity of science · Language precedes ontology

1.1 The Unity of Science

Moritz Schlick wrote in 1919: "*A philosophy of science does not hope to make the scientific disciplines sufficient and independent, but on the contrary to unify and unite them...Sub specie aeternitatis there is for him only one reality and one science.*"

In the early 1930s, Rolf Carnap formulated the three theses of the unity of science. The first of these asserts a certain unity of the language of science. This unity of the natural and social sciences is based on the same process of confirmation for all scientific statements, which gives them a character he calls 'intersubjective'; this is based on the ordinary language of observational data, enriched by the introduction of the concept of disposition, which bases its capacities on empirical foundations.

The second is a monistic thesis which considers that the sciences are reducible to each other in the sense of explanation, a thesis which is encouraged by the first partial successes of reduction then underway between chemistry and physics, from biology to chemistry and physics, and from psychology to neurophysiology.

The third thesis is that of the methodological unity of the sciences. Despite many differences in their investigative techniques, all branches of science support their theories in a manner that is ultimately very similar, deducing from them implications that are then subjected to the test of experiment or observation.

L. Karhausen, *The Fragility of Philosophy of Medicine*, Philosophy and Medicine 147, https://doi.org/10.1007/978-3-031-41633-0_1

The unity of science, according to Claudine Tiercelin, professor at the Collège de France, comes from the fact that scientific theories discover a world that is already structured, which is not constituted by our knowledge: if the scientific method leads to convergence, it is because it is constrained by reality [10].

1.2 The Disunity of Science [11]

Recent philosophy of science has been marked by a strong wave of support for heterodox views on the nature and ambitions of natural science. The themes of this new wave are the disunity of science, the autonomy of the individual sciences, anti-reductionism, and anti-fundamentalism. The Vienna Circle hoped to guarantee objectivity, rationality, truth, the possibility of knowledge in science, even going so far as to think that there was a methodology without content, so that knowledge and objectivity could be guaranteed. But we no longer have good reason to believe in this content-free methodology: there is hardly any methodology that is not uncertain.

Reductionism goes far beyond the realm of experience: it increasingly resembles a dogma which, moreover, is based on a somewhat outmoded metaphysical determinism. Can a biological phenomenon be exhaustively reduced to physico-chemical processes without residue? Biological phenomena are so complex that the idea of a complete explanation seems like a mirage. Explanations in science apply to certain aspects of a phenomenon, and they are never more than partial and limited.

The Stanford school of philosophy is characterized by pluralism, particularism, and interest in practice, as well as skepticism about the 'big system', which relies on long arguments and noble generalizations.

John Dupré advocates epistemological pluralism: there are many ways of certifying a scientific belief as knowledge, and there are many types of knowledge [12].

According to Alexander Rosenberg, the complexity of biological systems exceeds our ability to theorize for example, there is no way to relate Mendelian principles to molecular generalizations [13]. Theories are statements about how things would behave according to idealized models of reality. The very purpose of science is to assemble the best patchwork of local and phenomenological theories and laws, each characterized by its own field of application.

Nancy Cartwright also pointed out the increasing disunity that characterizes the sciences in general and consequently the medical sciences. Nancy Cartwright said that she does not know whether nature is disunified, but she would not find it reasonable to build a whole scientific methodology on the assumption that it must be unified. "*I think that knowledge of how the world should be, should be very closely related to knowledge of how the world is, and that big inductive leaps are hazardous, and we should be very careful about them... Personally, I am very suspicious of arguments that begin with things must be so and so, because...*"

Science as we know it is 'glittery'. Its picture of the world is a mosaic in which different aspects of the world, different systems, are represented by narrowly focused theories or models that are largely disconnected from each other. According to

Nancy Cartwright, the best explanation for this disunity in our representation of the world is a disunity of the world itself: rather than being governed by a small set of strict fundamental laws, events unfold according to a patchwork of principles covering all aspects of the world, each of which lacks total omnipotence with the possibility of anomic indeterminism at its edges. Nancy Cartwright is part of a whole movement of ideas that promotes the theme of the recent collapse of perceptions of distinct boundaries between science and non-science and between scientific disciplines.

Nancy Cartwright has been an important leader of this new wave: she rejects the received idea that everything that is explained is explained by universal generalizations or probabilistic generalizations [14].

She sees explanations as attributions of capabilities, which have nothing to do with universal generalizations. Capabilities are fundamental, not laws. Science then becomes less orderly. We assemble different pieces of theory to build models of real-life systems, and the method used to do this is by no means deductive. We know the capabilities of different kinds of characteristics, we know a series of situations in which we know explicitly what those capabilities will lead to. We think that the description of capabilities is universal, which is true, but it can in no way be translated into a modalized universal generalization. It must be seen as a capability statement that operates in a very different way from any of these laws as they are traditionally conceived.

All laws, in the sense of regularities, are generated by some mechanism, which deploys and exploits capacities, places them in the right circumstances, in the right connections with each other, keeps the whole thing stable enough, protects it and makes it work, and then we can see regularities appear. Most of these mechanisms are created by us. Little of what happens in the natural world is systematically governed, and it takes enormous effort under background conditions before regular and repeatable behavior is achieved. One of the reasons Nancy Cartwright likes to think in terms of capabilities is that it allows us to account for the fact that we have real scientific knowledge even in the case where there are no regularities. Acorns have the capacity to grow into oak trees. That oak tree in the garden came from an acorn that we planted there 20 years ago. There are many singular and true causal statements like that that go along with the ability to give birth to oaks without there being any regularity in what would happen repeatedly in all the circumstances where an oak or acorn would be planted.

In sum, Nancy Cartwright believes that there is positive evidence that nature is disunited: there are pockets of things that are quite distinct from each other and that behave in a regular enough way for us to understand them.

1.3 Nancy Cartwright, *Technè* and Possibilities

Aristotle in the Nicomachean Ethics describes two forms of knowledge: *Epistemè* and *Technè*.

Epistemè is scientific knowledge. It is universal, context-independent, and based on a general analytical rationality. *Technè* is pragmatic, instrumental, context-dependent, production- and action-oriented, based on a practical instrumental rationality, and governed by a conscious intention.

Nancy Cartwright defends the ontological thesis that scientific knowledge is, in fact, a *technè*. She argues that much of our important scientific knowledge is knowledge how, not knowledge that; that many of our most useful principles are neither true nor false but rather, in Pierre Duhem's terms, 'symbolic representations' that we use to model, predict and navigate the world; that many of these symbolic representations are shorthand labels for our powers and practices to use them; that our scientific successes do not suggest that nature operates by laws fixing what happens, but rather that the world is full of possibilities that are not in our models, nor in our representation of the world: they are real.

"*Our research, however*, "Wittgenstein wrote," *is not directed at phenomena, but one might say, at the 'possibilities' of phenomena.*" [15]

Scientific knowledge is the ability to carry out epistemic activities, and scientific truth is pragmatic consistency. Cartwright recommends renouncing truth for much of what are called 'scientific principles'. Not that these principles are wrong. Rather, they are not candidates for truth or falsity. Many of them make no claims at all. They are merely symbolic representations.

The context-centered approach focuses, according to Cartwright, on the context in which policies are to be implemented on understanding the causal pathways to the targeted outcome that it enables. It aims to use the accumulated knowledge to improve predictions about the effectiveness of policies in a target population.

On the other hand, moods, and intentional attitudes such as hopes, pretense, grief, intention, compliance, require a context. Therefore, Wittgenstein expressed this by saying that these terms refer to "*patterns in the weaving of our life*" [16]. To describe a human action, one must describe not only what "*a man is doing now, but the whole din of human actions*" of which an individual action is part [17].

The rules of language games express the relationship of men to the world as well as a partial convention and define the agreement between these two constraints as both given and decided. They merge into practices as much as they govern them. All meaningful behaviour is ipso facto governed by rules. For Cartwright, our scientific image of the world is constructed from our scientific practices that are effective in interacting with it.

But where does the priority lie? On the side of the world or on the side of language? On the language side, for Cartwright and for Wittgenstein. Language has only the world as a reference [18], so that if the world were different, the forms of life and the language games would also be different [19]. On the other hand, if the language games were different, the world would be conceived differently because '*theme and language are in reciprocal action*' [20].

For Wittgenstein, language precedes ontology.

Chapter 2
Wittgenstein's Toolbox

Abstract According to Wittgenstein, we use words to refer to reality, but we use them in language games. Language is an instrument, and philosophy is not a theory but an activity. Concepts such as disease, health, function, normal, abnormal, or treatment, usually have a definitional structure, which implies that there is a common essential element with sufficient and necessary conditions in all cases in which we apply the same term. However, Wittgenstein argues that those concepts are in fact linked by a quorum of overlapping and intersecting similarities, all of which have no common characteristics. This is the philosophical idea made popular by Wittgenstein, known as *family resemblances.*

Users of language are not guided by some mental act. To explain phenomena, we do not need to appeal to problematic mental states of "meaning something by an expression", since we rely on the natural fact that we belong to speech communities and that we agree on a linguistic practice.

Keywords Essentialism · Wittgenstein's family resemblances · Language games · Meaning · Following a rule

In a brilliant review of the history of analytic philosophy [21], Juliet Floyd, Professor of Philosophy at Boston University writes: "*Half a century after his death, Wittgenstein has already entered a relatively small canon of the history of modern philosophy, and his work has oriented philosophers in a wide range of fields, for his writings are at the heart of the analytic tradition, while being deeply critical of some of its more entrenched errors about meaning, content and objectivity.*"

His work is usually divided into first and second periods (those of the *Tractatus Logico-Philosophicus* and the *Philosophical Investigations*, respectively), but some insert an intermediate period (the time of works such as *The Blue Notebook and The Brown Notebook*) and others want to add a final period after the others (consisting exclusively of *On Certainty*). However, even though there has been progress in his way of thinking, there is a great unity in these so-called periods since his late approach of philosophy is already present in some of his early writings [22].

L. Karhausen, *The Fragility of Philosophy of Medicine*, Philosophy and Medicine 147, https://doi.org/10.1007/978-3-031-41633-0_2

He is arguing against a powerful philosophical tradition, namely the theory that words get their meaning either by representing objects, or by being associated with ideas in the mind, or because there must be an essence that the word expresses.

It might seem that, according to Wittgenstein's second philosophy, we use words to refer to objects in the world, but we use them in language games, and our concept of 'the world' and the way we divide the world is already conditioned by the structure of our language.

There is a shift from seeing language as an image to language as a tool. The nature of a tool is that it can be used for several different tasks: "*Language is an instrument. Its concepts are instruments*" [23]. Philosophy is not a theory but an activity, i.e., a *technè*. The difference between science and philosophy is between two distinct forms of understanding: the theoretical and the non-theoretical. Scientific understanding is given by the construction and testing of hypotheses and theories; philosophical understanding, on the other hand, is decidedly theoretical. What we are interested in in philosophy is "the understanding that consists in seeing connections".

He writes that "*Philosophy is a struggle against the bewitchment of our understanding by the resources of language*" [24]. He adds that philosophical problems arise when "*language goes on holiday*", i.e., when a word no longer does the job for which it is designed. We must always eliminate the intellectual confusions created by our inevitable urge to misunderstand the character of language.

What follows is a list of some of the main features of his late philosophy that are relevant to medical thinking.

2.1 Grammar

Wittgenstein goes against a long philosophical tradition dating back to Plato when he defends the idea at the heart of his philosophy that language precedes ontology.

One could say, with Antonia Soulez, that the only vein of Witttgenstein's philosophy is the discernment and elucidation of grammar. Grammar refers to the intellectual task necessary for language to succeed, so that pre-structured speech acts allow words to become acts. For Wittgenstein, philosophy is a grammatical enterprise: "*Grammar says of a thing what kind of object it is.... The* ***essence*** *is expressed in grammar*" [25].

And Antonia Soulez adds: "*It is indeed the internalist preoccupation with the 'grammatical' that runs through the work like the red thread of a single reflection, despite the breaks and phases, and which makes it possible to say that there are not several Wittgensteins, but only one*" [26].

Grammar refers both to the constitutive rules of language and to the philosophical study of the tabulation of these rules, as well as to the norms of correct use of certain words, expressions, phrases, or propositions. What Wittgenstein means by grammar are the rules for the correct use of words in a language, not only in the narrow or superficial sense usually intended when we speak of grammar, but also, and more importantly, in a more fundamental or advanced sense. In philosophy, grammar is sometimes called *the conditions of assertability*. Grammar refers to the intellectual task necessary for language to succeed, so that pre-structured speech acts allow words to become acts.

In the Tractatus (3.325), Wittgenstein argues that in order to avoid philosophical confusion, it is necessary to use a sign language (*Begriffsschrift*) governed by a logical grammar or logical syntax.

In his later work, Wittgenstein treats natural languages as having something like such a grammar, seeing them as intrinsically logical. Confusion arises, he says, when philosophers do not respect the rules of their own language.

Wittgenstein needed a better word than 'logic' to capture this phenomenon. So, he chose the word 'grammar' to give a name to the actions, procedures, and logics inherent in what people say. Grammar refers to the intellectual tasks necessary for language to succeed: they are pre-structured in speech acts and enable words to become acts.

According to the standard interpretation, the (syntactic) form of an expression, which would correspond to its surface grammar, does not reflect the way an expression is used, which corresponds to its depth grammar. And only the latter is relevant for determining its meaning. To make the point clearer, the expressions "I have a pin" and "I have a pain" have very similar surface grammars, but the former means some form of property of a thing, while the latter does not (it is a first-person confession). Similarly, does the word 'health' refer to a thing in the way that the word 'water' does?

It is said that when Wittgenstein was asked by a don at Trinity College, Cambridge, what surface grammar and deep grammar have in common, he replied: "*Should one say, 'The Father, the Son and the Holy Spirit is one God' or 'The Father, the Son and the Holy Spirit are one God'? Is it a question of surface grammar or depth grammar?*" [27].

For Wittgenstein, grammar (or what he sometimes calls logical syntax) is thus the overall system of grammatical rules, constitutive rules that define our language by determining what it is logical to say. This conception of rules is functional, that is, whether a sentence depends on a grammatical rule depends on its role or function within our linguistic practice.

Wittgenstein linked the concept of the meaning of a word to its use. The meaning of a word is the sum of its possible uses. The use of a word is determined by the rules for its use which are constitutive of what he calls "grammar" [28]. The use of words is a practice governed by implicit, normative, and shared rules, which imply regularities in their use; there must be agreement in explanations of the meaning of words and agreement in judgements.

Words are acts, so if language is a rule-guided activity, a grammatical rule depends on its role in our linguistic practice and in the framework conditions that make the rules practicable. Language is action-centered- language is what it does. "I can use the word 'yellow'" is like "I know how to move the king in chess."

Wittgenstein rejects the point-by-point correspondence between a thought and the situation it concerns. He rejects the idea that the structure and content of our language are somehow fixed by correspondence with reality, a reality external to language. According to him, the rules of grammar are arbitrary since the purpose of grammar is not external to that of language [29]. "*So, there is something arbitrary in this system? Yes and no. It is akin to what is arbitrary and what is not arbitrary*" [30]. The autonomy or arbitrariness of grammar has the effect that grammar itself cannot be justified in any way without an obvious circularity or total meaninglessness, since the concept of justification is part of that very language.

A *grammatical* proposition is a proposition whose truth value depends exclusively on specific grammatical rules. For example, everybody has an extension. In contrast, an empirical proposition depends for its truth value partly on the rules of usage of the words in it (grammar), and partly on empirical data.

Most of the time, science is for Wittgenstein only a collection of factual hypotheses that have no grammatical importance and are therefore of little or no interest to philosophy. Their grammatical importance is independent of their truth or falsity: this results from the shift of philosophy from the question of truth to the question of meaning.

Logic represents the a priori order of the world, i.e., it is "*common to the world and to thought*" [31]. This a priori order of the world is something that, according to Wittgenstein, must be common to the world and to thought. But this raises a paradox, which is that thought can be what it is not [32]: "*What I used to call 'objects', simple, was simply what I could refer to without running the risk of their possible non-existence; that is, what one can talk about no matter what*" [33].

What seems to have to exist, is part of language. Wherever we have a kind of necessity, Wittgenstein refers it to grammar. On the one hand, grammar is something variable and it is cut off from any underlying connection with reality: it is autonomous. But on the other hand, the knowledge of grammar remains the knowledge of a harmony between thought and reality. Only, this harmony is ensured entirely on the side of language [34].

In short, philosophy deals with possibilities and not with facts: its investigations are grammatical and not factual. Philosophy never needs to wait for certain facts to be established. Wittgenstein writes: "*Philosophy is content to place everything before us, without explaining or deducing anything*" [35].

2.2 The Quorum of Language: Family Resemblances (*Familienähnlichkeit*) or Similarities (*Ähnlichkeit*)

All classical theories concerning the structure of concepts are developments of or reactions to the theory of concepts, such as, in medicine, the concept of disease, an individual instance of disease, health, function, aging, healing, normal, abnormal, or pathological, etc. According to this theory, a concept has a definitional structure, which implies that there must be a common element in all cases where we apply the same general term. To grasp the enormous significance of this idea, we need only read the discussion of beauty in Plato's dialogue, *The Great Hippias* [36].

This theory is called *monothetic* in contrast to a *polythetic* approach, which argues that notions used in everyday life, in science or in philosophy can in fact be linked by a quorum of overlapping and intersecting similarities, all of which have no common characteristics. This is the philosophical idea made popular by Ludwig Wittgenstein, known as *family resemblances* [37].

The theory of *family resemblance predicates* (FRP) or *family resemblance terms* is one of the cores from which Wittgenstein's entire second philosophy is organized. "*I can think of no better expression to characterize these similarities than 'family resemblances'; for the various resemblances between members of a family: build, features, eye colour, gait, temperament, etc. etc., overlap and intersect in the same way*" [38].

Wittgenstein introduced this idea to combat an *essentialist* understanding of concepts, i.e., to show that the unity of concepts is not guaranteed by the identification of a set of common characteristics. We tend to believe that there must be something *essential* to the various situations that can be included under a given concept, and that, otherwise, there would be nothing to hold the different occurrences of these words together, and language would be reduced to anarchy.

The advantage of the notion of family resemblances or similarity over definitions specifying common characteristics is not that it concerns similarities instead of essences; rather, it is that agreement is ensured not by appealing to definitions but by bringing together in practice various applications that are cross-similar and overlapping.

Medical concepts such "health", "disease", "function", "normal or abnormal" are examples of family resemblances.

By analogy with the way members of a family resemble each other, this is the kind of similarity shared by things classified into certain groups: each shares characteristics with many but not all the others, *and there are no necessary or sufficient conditions* for belonging to this classification.

Wittgenstein argued that many of our concepts are concepts of family resemblance. "*Don't think, look ... you will see nothing in common with all of them, but you will see resemblances, kinships, and you will see a whole series of them.*"

A well-known variant is that of the rope which "*does not derive its strength from any fibre passing from one end to the other, but from the fact that many fibres overlap*" [39]. To someone who would say: "Something is therefore common to all these formations, namely the disjunction of all these common properties", I would retort: "You are only playing with a word". You could just as well say: "*Something is running all along the thread—namely the uninterrupted overlapping of these fibres*" [40].

2.3 Language Games (*Sprachspiel*)

Wittgenstein's failure to obtain a satisfactory general theory of language led him to conclude that there is an indefinite variety of uses of language, of language games.

"*I shall also call 'language game'*," Wittgenstein wrote, "*the whole formed by language and the activities with which it is interwoven.*"

A language game is a universe of linguistic behaviour and is Wittgenstein's shorthand for a rule-guided practice in which many people participate. He uses the term for language and its uses in a broad sense, including the way our language influences the way we think and act. A language game is a whole, "*composed of language and the actions into which it is transformed*". In short, language games are about the meaning of words, i.e., their use, the multiplicity of their uses and their relation to an activity. This allows for a flexible and action-oriented perspective on language and words.

Each language game has its own grammar. It seems that it is in the multiple and indefinite forms of ordinary language, and not in the formal and unique language of logic, that philosophy tries to deliver the expression of thought. The different systems of rules that correspond to different language games and the multiplicity of grammars reflect the indefinite diversity of communication games.

In his discussion of games, he argues that it is not necessary for games to have anything in common. "*Consider ...the processes we call 'games' ... pawn games, card games, ball games, fighting games. What do they all have in common?—Don't say: there must be something common to all of them, otherwise they wouldn't be called "games"—but* ***look*** *if there is something common to all of them*" [41, 42].

The emphasis here is on the similarity of a language to a game: games are systems of behaviour governed by rules, and the rules vary with time and context. Language, according to him, is a range of games, each with its own pieces and its own rules. Wittgenstein then lists the games of language: commanding or requesting, conjecturing, forming, or examining hypotheses, inventing stories, expressing a feeling or emotion, thanking, greeting, praying. Some of these are ambiguous: if I say, "Can you pass me the salt?" there is, in principle, little ambiguity since I am at the table with guests. However, a person with autism and impaired executive function might, for example, answer "yes" but, while he or she understands the question and makes it known, does not carry it out. Yes, it is a fact that she can pass the salt! [43]

Medicine, as well as the various scientific disciplines and specialties, are language games, which aim at an ordered understanding of a limited area of the world. The medical language game is itself composed of many intersecting, overlapping and sometimes conflicting language games, such as asking questions, testing hypotheses, making a diagnosis, estimating the likely course of a disease, assessing risks, screening for disease, identifying causal factors, explaining disease processes, making therapeutic decisions, and so on.

Some describe the world or health problems, some express emotions as a patient might, some show sympathy or seek to persuade as in the doctor-patient relationship, some are used to gather information or establish hypotheses as in the process of diagnosis, to give orders as in therapeutic decisions, to translate one language into another, to sing nursery rhymes and so on. They are not totally arbitrary because "*language is an instrument. Its concepts are instruments*" [44].

"*The expression "language play" makes it clear that speaking a language is part of an activity or a way of life*" [45]. We learn the rules of language in a certain context, a certain representation of the world, what Wittgenstein calls forms of life.

2.4 Forms of Life (*Lebensform, Weltbild*) [46]

The uses of language are varied and intertwined with the various activities in which people are engaged: a language game should be seen as a "*form of life*", i.e., a general communicative behaviour: "*speaking a language is part of an activity, or a form of life*" [47]. Rush Rhees writes: "*Language goes hand in hand with a form of life*" [48].

The term 'form of life' is used by Wittgenstein for several purposes. First, he introduces it, along with 'language play', to 'emphasize the fact that speaking a language is part of an activity, or a form of life'. We should not assume that the nature of language can be understood independently of the activities in which the uses of language are embedded.

A parallel thought is expressed, but this time in relation to emotions, such as hope and grief. Hope and grief, agitation, or depression, are not mere occurrences in the mind, but are embedded in the world in which we live and act, including the use of language, and are not meant to exist in isolation [49].

A way of life consists of patterns of behaviour, together with the conceptual frameworks and natural human capacities that make that behaviour possible. It is our habits of doing things together, which gives them meaning and makes learning possible. The concept of "form of life" which emphasizes the interweaving of culture, worldview and language has a long tradition in German philosophy with Herder, Hegel, Von Humboldt, and Spengler.

For Wittgenstein, a form of life is a culture or social formation, the totality of common activities in which language games are embedded. He sees language as a form of life: languages interpenetrate our lives and activities at every moment. They are common practices on which the normativity of language is based. They are contingent, but not arbitrary.

"*If a lion could speak, we would not understand it*" [50] because the life form of a lion and its behavioural repertoire is too foreign to us. This is an expression of the difference between the human life form and that of non-human animals.

Moods and intentional attitudes such as hopes, pretense, grief, intention, compliance with rules require a certain context.

Therefore, Wittgenstein expressed this by saying that these terms refer to "*patterns in the weaving of our life*" [51].

2.5 Following a Rule

Rules, laws, and instructions are obviously important. All sorts of problems would arise if they did not have a clear meaning. All communication could break down if people could not reliably follow the rules of language, namely grammar.

Wittgenstein argues that for language to have meaning, its use must follow certain rules. Yet language is not everywhere limited by rules: no system is ever limited by rules. Rules are subject to different interpretations. A rule is a social practice, it is something we do and learn in society.

A person follows a rule if he or she always acts in the same way on the same type of occasion. The use of the word 'rule' and the use of the word 'same' are intertwined, just like the use of the word 'proposition' and the use of the word 'true'.

Moreover, the notion of following a rule is logically inseparable from the notion of error, i.e., a deviation from what is established as correct.

Following a rule thus raises the problem of the normativity of standards: how does a rule determine what counts as a correct or incorrect application? [52] A rule is a standard of correctness or rectitude. Applying a rule correctly does not mean doing what most people do, because rules could be misapplied by whole groups. There are no rules unless there is a practice of 'obeying' or 'going against' them. Internal relationships are affected by our normative activities: we teach and explain the rules, we criticize them, we justify them, and it is by reference to them that we characterize our actions [53].

Wittgenstein describes following a rule as a social practice because it is impossible to follow a rule privately. Some rule-guided activities such as buying, selling, doing mathematics, making a diagnosis, or treating a patient require the context of a social and historical way of life [54].

There is a difference between following a rule and acting according to a rule. If an agent follows a rule, this does not distinguish him or her from natural regularities such as the movement of the planets. But if an agent follows a rule, the rule must be part of the reason for acting and not its cause: he must intend to follow the rule [55].

"Is what we call 'following a rule' something that a single man could do once in his life?—This is a comment on the grammar of the expression "follow the rule". It is not possible for a rule to have been followed by one man only once ... Following a rule, passing on information, giving an order, playing a game of chess are customs (usages, institutions)" [56].

All sorts of problems can arise if rules, laws, and instructions have no clear meaning; if people cannot tell how to follow them, or whether someone has followed them or not.

A rule is abstract in such a way that the applications of the rule are not. The very literal meaning of a rule is, in a sense, impossible to specify. There could be an infinite number of circumstances in which a rule could be applied, and the rule itself will not say, at least explicitly, what to do in each case.

The rules of language games express the human relationship to the world as well as a partial convention and define the agreement between these two constraints as both given and decided. They merge into practices as much as they govern them. All meaningful behaviour is ipso facto governed by rules.

2.6 Saul Kripke: One of the Best Readings of Wittgenstein

Saul Kripke has produced an exceptionally clear and vivid account of the central argument of Wittgenstein's Philosophical Investigations. He does not claim that his version of the work is in any way faithful to Wittgenstein's intentions, which may not be sufficiently defined to be accurately rendered. Much of Wittgenstein's so-called later philosophy is here lucidly reformulated, integrated and made highly plausible [57].

Kripke's argument is based on a statement from the Philosophical Investigations: "*Our paradox was this: A rule could not determine any way of acting, since any way of acting can be made to agree with the rule: If everything can be made to agree with the rule, then everything can also contradict it. And so there would be neither agreement nor contradiction... So, there is an inclination to say: Any action that proceeds according to the rule is an interpretation. But we should only call "interpretation" the substitution of one expression of the rule for another*" [58].

It is natural to suppose that when we use a word or symbol in our language we are guided in its use by our understanding of its meaning, or of the concept it expresses, or of the rules or instructions for its use which we have mastered; that it is these things which tell us that it is correct to use the expression in this or that way, to apply it to this case. So, we seem to be invoking a fact of our mental life to explain our confidence in the correctness of our present use of the expression.

If we take this conception seriously, it seems that there is no guarantee that what we mean by an expression today is identical to what we meant by it in the past. The conclusion is that the very conception invoked in the argument, however natural it may seem, should not be taken seriously. It is illusory.

Kripke then confesses to a "strange feeling" when contemplating this conclusion. "*It seems as if all idea of meaning vanishes into thin air*". He wonders if it is possible to escape this skeptical conclusion by looking for an acceptable candidate for the role of fact, or mental element, which will constitute my meaning of this or that thing by an expression.

What is the solution?

First, we must abandon the chimerical idea that the user of language is guided by the mental fact in the light of which he judges that its application in a particular case is justified or correct.

There must be room for the idea of correct use. We are dealing with communities of language users, and the test of the correct use of an expression is the test of conformity to the use of an expression in each community. There must be publicly observable bases for the application of these expressions, which he calls 'criteria'. Hence the famous doctrine that expressions relating to internal processes need external criteria.

The great lesson of this view is that there is, philosophically speaking, nothing behind it, and that there is no need for something beyond or behind it to constitute a philosophical explanation. Although there may be biological, anthropological, cultural, and historical explanations, as far as the philosophical problem is concerned, we can simply rely on, or take as primitive, the great natural fact that we form speech communities, that we agree on a linguistic practice and so on. It is useless and misleading to appeal to problematic mental states of 'meaning something by an expression', to explain phenomena.

Chapter 3
Medicine

The difficulty in philosophy is to say no more than we know.
Wittgenstein

Abstract According to Wittgenstein, we use words to refer to reality, but we use them in language games. Language is an instrument, and philosophy is not a theory but an activity. Concepts such as disease, health, function, normal, abnormal, or treatment, usually have a definitional structure, which implies that there is a common essential element with sufficient and necessary conditions in all cases in which we apply the same term. However, Wittgenstein argues that those concepts are in fact linked by a quorum of overlapping and intersecting similarities, all of which have no common characteristics. This is the philosophical idea made popular by Wittgenstein, known as *family resemblances.*

Users of language are not guided by some mental act. To explain phenomena, we do not need to appeal to problematic mental states of "meaning something by an expression", since we rely on the natural fact that we belong to speech communities and that we agree on a linguistic practice.

Keywords Scientific philosophy · Diseases · Pregnancy · Abortion · Medically unexplained symptoms · Biological negativities · Fictitious diseases · Medicalization

"*Medicine is a curious discipline in some respects, for it is practically the only professional specialty that claims the titles of science and makes its judgement primarily in terms of prescriptive norms...*", wrote Joseph Margolis [59].

What distinguishes it from biology in the first place is what is pathological, i.e., all biological forms of physical or mental suffering, causes of mortality, and the means to correct, prevent or explain them. This notion is not scientifically definable, as it is not defined by its descriptive, cognitive, and performative nature. Medicine is a system that is essentially concerned with the identification and correction of biological, physical, and mental negativities, as well as—whether these are present, possible, or not—a precautionary and preventive approach at the level of individuals, higher animals, and the population. Many of these situations represent diseases

L. Karhausen, *The Fragility of Philosophy of Medicine*, Philosophy and Medicine 147, https://doi.org/10.1007/978-3-031-41633-0_3

or syndromes, but an important if not a major fraction in humans consists of isolated, repetitive new sets of signs or symptoms, which are generally either difficult to explain or medically unjustified.

"*Medicine,*" writes John Margolis, "*is a professionalized specialty concerned with a limited range of general prudential goals: just those that depend, minimally, on the state of the body being adjusted to allow, at that point, the achievement of those goals or, by extension, the analogous state of the mind or person. Like law, medicine is a prudential art. But where law is concerned with the order between individuals and aggregates, medicine is concerned with the ability to use our bodies, our minds and ourselves as effective instruments, insofar as all our projects depend on a particular personal effort... Clearly, to define medicine in this way is also to provide a basis for multiple conceptions of medical standards*" [60].

The question of the nature of medicine is not an internal problem of the medical discipline. Medicine is a set of activities but talking about medicine is not a medical activity. In other words, talking about medicine is external to medicine, but internal to philosophy.

"*The philosophy of science,*" writes Dr. R. S. Downie, "*is a flourishing discipline, as is moral philosophy. Medicine, which combines elements of both, has not received as much attention. This is partly a result of the attention paid to medical ethics, which has obscured the need for a philosophical foundation for medicine*" [61]. A bastard medicine is at once naturalistic and normativist, reductionist and holistic, realist and pragmatist, phenomenalist and instrumentalist, objective and subjective, between science and technique, language and action, facts and values, empiricism and conventions, what is and what should be, and it is always on the edge of naturalistic paralogism by its language that is both descriptive and prescriptive. It is also unbreakable and cannot be dismembered into science and practice, *technè* and *epistemè*, at the risk of serious confusion. It follows that medical science considers the world in terms of hybrid concepts that have two dimensions: they have one foot in the world and a second in values. Medicine is a science, but medical theory and medical language must also be seen as instrumental in controlling disease or harmful conditions: they have instrumental value because they have value to another end. Truth and falsity are then reduced to conventional positive or negative standards. Pragmatism is sympathetic to instrumentalism, since it assumes that any belief is a mere acceptance into the system deemed most useful.

Factual or scientific beliefs do not guide action, they are neutral. It is the combination of cognitive knowledge and intention that engages an architect in designing and carrying out his work project. Medical concepts are intersections of factual and intentional markers in which the implicit need for health intervention is inherent in the actual or potential deleterious quality of pathological features. Despite this, medical statements are not properly dual, i.e., consisting of factual statements about signs and symptoms on the one hand and valuing assertions about needs on the other: the two are intrinsically linked to each other and merge. All in all, medical terms are what Sir Bernard Williams has called thick terms, whereby the thoughts and judgements expressed by these statements, on the one hand, are candidates for truth and falsity ('*world-guided*') and, on the other, provide reasons for action ('*action-guiding*') [62].

Medicine has no clear boundaries, and it is impossible to conceptually separate medicine from other practices by referring to its so-called goals [63], because these goals are shared with several other disciplines. It is part of that second way of describing the world that Immanuel Kant spoke of, that which concerns our interests, what is biologically right or wrong, and which makes it possible to guide our actions, what Aristotle and Nancy Cartwright call a *technè*.

Medicine is what Wittgenstein calls an institution, i.e., a collective model of self-referential activity [64]. Medicine is defined by the diversity of topics addressed by doctors and health systems. This means that invoking normative categories is an act of participation in a self-referential practice with no independent source of justification. An attempt to justify a 'must' can only lead us back to medical practice itself.

To define medicine is either to say what the essence of medicine really is (a real definition) or to say what the meaning of the word "medicine" is (a "nominal definition"). In the latter case, it may be to describe the sense in which the word is currently used (a descriptive or dictionary definition) or to prescribe a meaning for that word (a prescriptive or stipulative definition).

Wittgenstein rejected the explanation of concept acquisition in terms of abstraction, i.e. the interpretation of all words as *nouns* [65] carrying an *essence:* one acquires a concept by acquiring the relevant linguistic competence, by being raised to use the word according to the rules of practice implicitly accepted by the members of one's linguistic community: "*When philosophers use a word—"knowledge", "being", "object", "I", "proposition", "name"—and strive to capture the essence of the thing in question, one must always ask: is this word actually used in this way in the language where it has its place of origin?*" [66].

Wittgenstein concludes that in most cases, the meaning of a word can be defined as follows: *meaning is use* [67]. And this brings us back to medical practice, far from philosophical abstractions and sociological and historical considerations.

What are the objects of medical activities?

- Defining and identifying *diseases* and *syndromes,* i.e., categorizing them, is a fraction of health service practice. Diseases are vague, unstable, difficult to circumscribe, uncertain and conservative conventions that describe biological, organic, or mental pathological processes experienced by a creature, recognized by medical science, and which have varying degrees of severity or mortality. The categorization and classification of diseases is subject to modification, rectification, and reworking; they generally have uncertain boundaries and are rarely delimited entities. The notion of disease is therefore not the starting point of medicine, but one of its end points.
- A second important fraction consists of the so-called iceberg of explained, unexplained or unexplainable symptoms, the MES (*medically unexplained symptoms*) [68]. The world of medicine is like the starry sky: there are an unlimited number of stars, and a finite number of constellations or diseases.
- Then there are phenomena that do not belong to biological negativities such as pregnancy, childbirth, menstruation, menopause, sterility, disabilities, short stature, sport, the ten principles of cosmetic practice, reconstructive surgery,

baldness, contraceptive methods, abortion, euthanasia, therapeutic ageing, artificial fertilization, and surrogate mothers—but which represent common interventions in medicine.
- A fourth fraction, which manifests itself as a high demand for care in the absence of a need for care, is imperatively imposed on the health system: it is constituted, for example, by the promotion of *'fictitious diseases'*, transmitted by word of mouth or by the media—to the great displeasure of doctors—such as multiple personality syndrome, electromagnetic hypersensitivity, fear of glyphosate, multiple chemical sensitivity or Gulf War syndrome, as well as, probably, the hysteria syndrome described by Charcot and Freud [69].
- Long-standing concerns about what the World Health Organization defines as a public health problem: "violence" against a person, group, or community [70].
- Next are new ideas in medical research, such as genetic therapies or the use of stem cells and their derivatives, a therapy that promotes the repair of diseased, dysfunctional, or injured tissue. It is the next chapter in organ transplantation and uses cells instead of donor organs, which are in limited supply.
- "*Man is something to be overcome*", wrote Nietzsche. Enhancement is a concept that defines improvements to the human organism through non-therapeutic or perfective procedures in the fields of genetics, neuroscience, pharmacology, and physiology, from optimizing the functioning of human capacities to cosmetic modifications or the medicalization of unhappiness. Jonathan Glover [71] has provided the most comprehensive and effective discussion of the ethical, political, social, and medical dimensions of enhancing and overcoming human biological boundaries.

Here we find the difficult, experimental, and still poorly understood issue of care—especially pediatric care—for gender dysphoria and its ethical aspects. It is likely that many of the disagreements in the medical philosophy literature stem from the fact that certain conceptual distinctions have been introduced which may seem legitimate to philosophers, but which could be circumvented if one is interested in medical practice. "*It is astonishing,*" wrote William James, "*how many philosophical disputes collapse into insignificance as soon as they are subjected to this simple test of tracing a concrete consequence*" [72]. Medicine tells us how physicians intuitively organize nature, not how nature is organized.

In his pamphlet *Medical Nemesis* [73], Ivan Illitch suggests that medicine tends to appropriate various aspects of life, including pain, ageing, death, patient expectations and curative and preventive therapies. The pathologizing of normal life events and the conversion of risks into diseases extend medical concepts outside the medical domain, with therapeutics spilling over into culture. This unattainable goal runs the risk of medicalizing features and difficulties in our lives that are not within the competence and remit of medicine. At the beginning of the twenty-first century, social factors have tended to shift the line between the notions of "normal" and "pathological" and to change a condition from that of a social deviance to that of a disease, especially in behavioural disorders. Alcohol abuse, addiction, suicide, certain forms of delinquency, menopause, pregnancy, induced abortion, euthanasia, pedophilia, maladjustment are now labelled as medical.

Ivan Illitch has argued, in a 'Rousseauist' tradition, that society is so unhealthy that it knowingly threatens the survival of humanity and knowingly produces much of the serious and fatal disease in individuals. But these threats to the survival of the species are outside the scope of medical care. The fact that humanity is destroying its "ecological niche" is true, but is not within the scope of medicine, except insofar as it has public health consequences, such as the risk of global epidemics or potentially fatal viral diseases, or climate change. Any condition that leads to limited incapacity is a matter for medicine, but where to start? Perhaps Illich simply wanted to highlight the illegitimate invasion of non-medical social concerns into the field of medicine and the efforts to move medicine away from its core mission. The philosophical question of the limits of medicine is therefore not without interest, but philosophy can only observe and describe. It is medical practice—and to some extent public opinion—that inevitably tends to expand the boundaries of medicine.

Sometimes the *courts create a disease* or a risk factor that does not exist. The US courts have ruled that Bayer, the German agrochemical giant, must compensate people who, after using Roundup, developed non-Hodgkin's lymphoma, even though the causal relationship between these two events is known to be wrong: there is hardly a necessary or sufficient causal relationship between glyphosate and any disease.

Risk factors such as smoking, alcohol and drug abuse, environmental exposures, air pollution, occupational hazards, contamination of the food chain by various chemicals or wastes, the consequences of overpopulation and climate change, wars and forms of social violence have given rise to new or changing public health-related prudential concerns as medical and public health practices have expanded their scope and entered the territory of public policy. Thus, prudential needs should define the boundaries of medicine.

However, the practice of medicine is a set of practices, a *family of life forms*—diagnosis, treatment, prevention, screening—that are not necessarily consistent with each other. A diagnostic liver puncture may lead to an abdominal hemorrhage and anticoagulant treatment in a patient with atrial fibrillation may cause a fatal brain hemorrhage. Medicine is a patchwork of specialties and subspecialties that are constantly being orchestrated and divided into clinical microsystems between which communication is likely to be problematic. It is not uncommon for communication to be difficult or awkward between a general practitioner and a tertiary care hospital.

David Aron in his book about the complexity of medical practice and research, about clinical forms of life that are not always compatible with each other, insists that understanding complex systems can greatly assist a doctor in coping with the many challenges and facets of his experience [74].

Chapter 4
Diseases, Injuries, and Disabilities

Abstract There is an essentialist and a non-essentialist quorum view of disease. There are three philosophical theories of illness: naturalism, normativism, and a hybrid model. Medicine is both descriptive and prescriptive. Diseases are biological negativities; they are medical constructs; they have specific causes, a natural history, and they need medical intervention. Diseases may have genomic biomarkers. Diseases are classified into categories. Is ageing a disease?

Keywords Disease, injury, disability · Need for treatment · Naturalism · Normativism · Hybrid models · Natural kinds · Causal and descriptive diseases · Natural history · Classification of diseases · Ageing · Non-existing diseases · Essentialism · Vagueness · The language quorum

Diseases, unlike injuries and disabilities, are processes. Since Thomas Sydenham, it has been accepted that these psycho-physiological processes fall into certain classes or species, called "disease entities". The criteria used for the classification of diseases predominantly include information on prevention and treatment. To call something a disease entity is to say that it is an example of the kind of psychophysiological process that people want to be able to prevent or interrupt. It follows that disease is a value-bearing concept.

The definition of illness is the subject of endless debate and discussion. To be ill is to be a victim of a value-laden process that involves a commitment to medical intervention, the attribution of the role of patient, and the enlistment of health professionals in the action [75]. More precisely, a person who is the object of a process or condition such that he or she experiences or risks suffering infirmity, harm, physical or mental suffering, an inability to do certain things [76], or the possibility of dying, is then medically ill.

Certain pairs of terms that are the cornerstone of medical doctrines, such as normal/abnormal or normal/pathological, health/disease, life/death, show a clear asymmetry. "*We are pain, not the absence of pain*" wrote Schopenhauer [77]. "*Often it is the abnormal that sheds light on the normal*" wrote John Austin [78].

L. Karhausen, *The Fragility of Philosophy of Medicine*, Philosophy and Medicine 147, https://doi.org/10.1007/978-3-031-41633-0_4

To be ill is essentially to be a victim of a pathological process. What is pathological is conceptually prior to what is normal. Spinoza's adage *Omnis determinatio est negatio* is the most famous of modern statements about the negative and has been fruitful in terms of outcomes [79]. Once under the care of health services, a sick person becomes a patient, and illness becomes socially an absence or negation of health: illness ceases to be the property of a person, but becomes an entity separate from the person [80].

Carolyne Whitbeck wrote that: "*Diseases such as forest fires, car accidents, as well as injuries and disabilities, are the type of things that people wish they could control in some way. With all such things, we eliminate, terminate, diminish, etc. these things, and that is why we see the evaluation involved as negative*" [81].

4.1 Injury and Trauma

"Injury", "trauma" or "wound" are all synonyms. Any process triggered by the infliction of an injury is either a healing process, a pathological process (e.g., staphylococcal infection) or a combination of both. In its descriptive content, the concept of injury is endowed with values, as is the concept of disease.

4.2 Impairment and Disabilities

An impairment is a persistent psychophysiological abnormality, which people wish to prevent or correct because it interferes with the carrier's ability to do what people want and expect to be able to do.

4.3 Disease

Diseases can be classified as congenital or acquired, acute or chronic, iatrogenic, or idiopathic. They may have external or internal causes. There are many categories of diseases, including infectious diseases, hereditary diseases, deficiency diseases and physiological diseases. Patients may have a disease without knowing it. Conversely, patients may feel ill and suffer from a disease when they have none, such as electromagnetic hypersensitivity.

If we rigidly assume that medical diagnostic categories are fixed entities, we will not recognize variations of a previously undescribed disease, or even an entirely new disease. A condition that is considered a disease today might be considered a variant of normal in the future, and vice versa.

But disagreements over ordinary words such as "disease" are not based on "definitions" or facts. Rather, they arise from the way these words are treated in the medical language game. This means that appeals to "standard definitions", or to facts and science, are completely misplaced.

The real question is not whether a particular definition is wrong, but whether the very attempt to fix a rigid set of essential characteristics is, as Wittgenstein would have argued, misguided. For Wittgenstein, the meaning of a word or sign is not an entity that determines its use. A word becomes meaningful not by its association with an object, but by a usage that obeys a rule, i.e., its meaning depends on the way it is used: "*For a large class of the cases in which it is used—but not for all of them—the word 'meaning' can be explained in the following way: The meaning of a word is its use in language*" [82].

What do diseases like pneumonia, panic disorder, impacted wisdom teeth, rheumatoid arthritis, male impotence, primary immune thrombocytopenia, schizophrenia, Covid 19, gastric ulcer, disability, restless leg syndrome, Munchausen's syndrome, or old age have in common? Do they have something in common and must they have something in common?

It appears that diseases have no essence, but form a set loosely assembled by certain pathophysiological events that express themselves as signs and symptoms deemed undesirable. No characteristic is necessary or essential for something to be what we call a disease. What is crucial is that the links between pathophysiology, objective clinical signs, subjective symptoms, and their deemed undesirability, are not logically determined.

The eminent epidemiologist Archie Cochrane [83] has called these "*group concepts*" based on what has sometimes been described as the quorum feature of language: a group of characteristics associated with a disease name is such that they need not all be present; any one of them may be absent if some of them are present; the more of them there are, the more comfortable we feel about applying the term.

Diseases are linked together not by an essence expressed in a definition, but because they form what Rorty calls *a web of beliefs* [84]. To know a disease, one must know how society or doctors view diseases, and this knowledge is derived from experience, not from definition [85]. Diseases, if we follow Wittgenstein, are forms of representation; it is a misuse of the term 'meaning' to regard their meaning as the object they denote. The meaning of a word is not any object, but its use according to grammatical rules.

"*In practice,*" writes Wittgenstein, "*if you were asked which phenomenon is a criterion of definition and which is a symptom, you would in most cases be unable to answer this question, except by making an arbitrary ad hoc decision. It may be convenient to define a word by taking a phenomenon as a defining criterion, but we will easily be persuaded to define the word by means of what we first use as a symptom. Doctors will use names for diseases without ever deciding which phenomena should be taken as criteria and which as symptoms; and this is not necessarily a deplorable lack of clarity. For remember, we do not generally use language according to strict rules—nor have we been taught by means of strict rules. Instead, in our discussions, we constantly compare language to a calculation that takes place according to precise rules*" [86].

Moreover, in the case of "disease", the singular-universal distinction is important and manifests itself on two levels: two different things that are both of a certain type are said to be tokens of a certain type. Disease as a concept is a type, a universal, while diseases as clinical entities are tokens, particulars. Clinical entities are then universals that are instantiated by patients.

"*Compare the grammar of this word*," Wittgenstein writes, "*when it denotes a particular kind of disease, with that of the expression 'Bright's disease' when it means 'the disease that Bright has'. I will characterize this difference by saying that in the first case the word 'Bright is an index within the complex noun 'Bright's disease'; in the second case I will say that it is an argument of the function 'the disease of x*" [87].

The term "disease" in medical grammar applies either to the concept of disease, or to the various specific categories of disease, or to the disease of a given patient. Diseases involve the grouping of sick people into categories that are considered useful in managing their condition or in understanding the circumstances that led to it [88]. They are variously referred to as diseases, conditions, ailments, illnesses, clinical entities, disease entities, syndromes or nosological entities. The great clinician W. Osler of the early twentieth century wrote: "*Variability is the law of life, and as no two faces are alike, no two bodies are alike, and no two individuals react in the same way and behave in the same way under the abnormal conditions we know as diseases*" [89].

Now, if the notion of "disease" is one of the main junctures in medicine, its usefulness is in no way altered by its imprecision. Following Ludwig Wittgenstein, by analogy with the way members of a family resemble each other, it is the kind of similarity that diseases and their categorizations share: there are no necessary and sufficient conditions for belonging to these categories. Since disease has no essence, for a given disease, each patient shares characteristics with many other patients, but not with all. The disease categories are not mutually exclusive and are not jointly exhaustive [90].

Even worse, having two serious infectious diseases, for example HIV and TB, is worse than having only one: it is worse because the effects are not additive but synergistic. These synergistic effects are called *syndemias* [91]. In a diabetic patient, hypertension is a clinically concordant comorbidity because it is part of the same overall pathophysiological risk profile, and its treatment goes hand in hand with diabetes. Epidemiology indicates that comorbidity is quite common.

Moreover, the clinical entities of the manuals may overlap, and not only in the case of mental disorders. For example, Alzheimer's disease is a neurocognitive disorder characterized by beta-amyloid deposits and neurofibrillary tangles in the cerebral cortex and subcortical grey matter. Lewy body dementia is also a neurocognitive disorder characterized by cellular inclusions called Lewy bodies in the cytoplasm of cortical neurons. Lewy bodies are sometimes present in Alzheimer's disease, and patients with Lewy body dementia may have neurofibrillary tangles [92].

The same disease, Down's syndrome, may be due to two different causes, either a trisomy or a translocation of chromosome 21. If the concept of disease is both

historical [93] and cultural [94], the clinical entities that constitute it are medical: they are created, modified, divided, abandoned, adjusted, or rewritten to meet the needs of medicine or public health, as well as influenced, i.e., expanded or created by the pharmaceutical [95] and food industries [96].

In sum, the idea that in order to understand the meaning of a general term, one must find elements common to all its applications has undermined philosophical research; for not only has it failed to produce any results, it has also led philosophy to reject as irrelevant the concrete cases, which alone could have helped it to understand the use of the general term. Wittgenstein therefore advocates proceeding here by considering the way in which any claim to or denial of knowledge is made, and that this can be done by enumerating instances of known things [97].

4.4 The Nature of Disease

Jeremy Simon suggests that there may not be a unitary concept of disease, but rather a family of related concepts. We can think of disease as an object of medical research, as a state or process that legitimizes treatment, as a state that implies that a patient can legitimately enter the 'sick role', and so on. Simon believes that separate philosophical approaches may be needed for each of these varied, though related, concepts [98].

Sedgwick writes: "*Apart from the meaning which man voluntarily attaches to certain conditions, there are no diseases or ailments in nature.... Are there not infections and contagious bacilli? Are there not definite and objective lesions in the cellular structures of the human body? Are there not bone fractures, fatal tissue ruptures, malignant multiplications of tumour growth? Yet these natural events do not—before the human social meanings we attribute to them—constitute ailments, ailments, or diseases*" [99].

Informed clinicians are aware that diagnostic categories are only concepts justified and based on whether they provide a useful framework for intellectually organizing and explaining the complexity of clinical experience to make predictions about outcomes and guide treatment decisions. However, once a diagnostic concept has come into use, it tends to become reified, and there is a tendency to assume that it is an entity. This is where the endless philosophical debates between normativists and naturalists begin.

Disease is a bit like a "weed". A weed is simply an unwanted plant, a quack grass, a daisy, a dandelion; no botanical characteristics are necessary or sufficient to define it.

Dying is not a disease, but if men tended to be immortal, it would be. Pregnancy could very easily be considered an infection, and if what we consider normal aging could easily be avoided for an interval four times longer than a normal life span, "normal aging" could be treated as a sign of disease.

Concepts belong to those who make them work. The term ‘disease’ belongs to the grammar of medical language, even though the idea of disease is part of ordinary language.

Many definitions have been proposed that are the subject of endless controversy. Some years ago, in a book entitled *What is a disease?* Several authors have attempted to arrive at a kind of definition [100]. What was surprising was that each author had his own definition and managed to defend it. But none of them tried to find out why they disagreed with each other.

Experts from different disciplines (e.g., anatomy, biochemistry, genetics) may have very different views on the naturalness of the boundaries of accepted disease categories, and categories that seem natural at one time may no longer be so in the light of new knowledge.

“*In practice*,” writes Wittgenstein, “*if you were asked which phenomenon is a criterion of definition and which is a symptom, you would in most cases be unable to answer this question, except by making an arbitrary ad hoc decision. It may be convenient to define a word by taking a phenomenon as a defining criterion, but we will easily be persuaded to define the word by means of what we first use as a symptom. Doctors will use names for diseases without ever deciding which phenomena should be taken as criteria and which as symptoms; and this is not necessarily a deplorable lack of clarity. For remember, we do not generally use language according to strict rules—nor have we been taught by means of strict rules. Instead, in our discussions, we constantly compare language to a calculation that takes place according to precise rules*” [101].

The definition of illness is the subject of endless debate and discussion, as we have seen above. A sick person is either a person who feels like one, or a person who is defined as such by society, or a person who is recognized as such by the health services. The existential quest is not purely mental or emotional but concerns our bodies which are the very expression of this demand, of our own integrity and self-concept. People subscribe to prudential values—avoiding death, prolonging life, satisfying desires, ensuring security of person and body and property.

To be sick is to be a victim of a biological negativity that involves a commitment to medical intervention, the attribution of the role of sickness, and the enrolment in the action of health professionals [102]. Specifically, a person who is the object of a process or condition such that he or she experiences or is at risk of suffering infirmity, harm, physical or mental suffering, inability to do certain things [103], or the possibility of dying, is then medically ill.

Even an autosomal dominant genetic disease such as acute intermittent porphyria (of which Cochrane himself was a sufferer) shows an asymmetric but unimodal distribution of total fecal porphyrin among the 150 members of a family in which there had been a case. In other words, the multimodality implied by clinical descriptions is often the result of selective biases inherent in clinical or hospital samples, rather than their actual distribution in the general population. Most diseases are quantitative and present us with a scalar and continuous distribution of attributes or characteristics. Disease is a family resemblance term, and no clear boundaries are imposed.

Diseases as a process are a whole spectrum, a range of symptoms that often but not always coexist, with significant variation from patient to patient, a continuum in all degrees and degrees of severity, not a dichotomy as abnormal features manifest themselves on a continuum that extends to normal features.

Wittgenstein's emphasis on '*in-between cases*' is important. Philosophy must be done on the ground: we must reason from something insular, not general [104]. Concrete examples are always the backdrop. It is like proceeding to "*a series of examples*" where problems are solved, and difficulties eliminated [105].

However, there are certain types of words that totally resist family resemblance. Words with technical or scientific connotations often succeed. This phenomenon is called rigidity. Hydrogen peroxide or H^2O^2 cannot have more than one meaning in the language game. Causal diseases are rigid concepts because they are defined by a single cause. Tuberculosis is a disease defined by Koch's bacillus. We are therefore either sometimes in a situation of prescribing this concept in the case of causal diseases, or in a situation of locating its meaning in the general case of diseases.

Except for causal entities, there is an ultimately imperceptible gradation between the sick and the non-diseased. Most diseases present us with a smooth and continuous distribution of attributes: their manifestations gradually degrade in a linear order into "normal" characteristics and there is no point at which a dividing line can be drawn, except in a very arbitrary way.

In addition, some disease processes may be distinct, such as Tay-Sachs disease or thalassemia, and genetically inherited diseases with high penetrance; they are separate from other diseases or from the normal population if the differences between them, whether qualitative or quantitative, are discontinuous. A discrete entity, such as Balkan nephropathy, may still be indistinguishable if its prevalence is low and the mean distribution of its manifestations is close to that of normal creatures: in this case the disease entity remains hidden in the normal distribution curve.

There are no simple patients: all patients are complex. The complexity of the patient is manifested in many interactions, in the consequences and interdependence of these interactions which are not always predictable. When they are predictable in a patient with asthma and diabetes, treatment of asthma with glucocorticoids such as prednisone for its anti-inflammatory effects leads to worsening of diabetes due to the hyperglycemic effects of these drugs.

Disease has a central place in medical practice even if it is not its focus. Medical thinking emerged centuries before the first conceptualization of the notion of "disease" was developed.

4.5 The Philosophy of Medicine and the Problem of Disease

Today, philosophers are still faced with the need to better define the concept of disease and how diseases can and should be classified into types. On another note, 'disease' is a term used primarily by doctors and health care personnel, so its medical use is likely to be remote from the different philosophical understandings in which it is understood.

There are now several philosophical theories of illness. Ereshefsky proposes to group them into three categories: naturalistic, normativist and hybrid [106].

(i) **Naturalism**

Naturalism is the theory that the concept of disease reflects an objective reality about cells, organs, or systems of function or dysfunction. The grouping of sick people involves the search for categories that are somehow natural. The principle behind these claims is that a classification system should be evaluated in terms of how close it comes to the Platonic ideal of cutting up nature at its joints [107].

A realist position accounts for its meaning in terms of its *truth conditions.*

According to J.G. Scadding: "A disease is the sum of abnormal phenomena exhibited by a group of living organisms in association with a common specific characteristic or set of characteristics by which they differ from the norm of their species so as to be biologically disadvantaged".

Echoing Scadding [108], Christopher Boorse has developed and defended the contemporary naturalistic theory that is also the most widely discussed. Boorse defines disease as: "a type of internal state that is either an impairment of normal functional capacity, i.e., a reduction of one or more functional capacities below its usual effectiveness, or a limitation of functional capacity, caused by environmental agents" [109]. Health is then the absence of disease.

Boorse argues that diseases are recognizable against the objective backdrop of species-typical function, a concept borrowed from Scadding. The epistemological core of Boorse's theory of disease is statistical, and the determination of species specificity is supposed to be empirical. Indeed, Boorse labelled his form of naturalism 'biostatistical theory'. Biological dysfunction is then both necessary and sufficient to define the disease.

Boorse introduces a distinction between disease and illness. He recognizes that the concept of illness is normative, while that of disease is not, so that illnesses are particular, and diseases are universal. Illness is a sub-category of disease. Disease is then a professional and medical term, while illness concerns the patient's perspective [110].

Secondly, Boorse recognizes that the attribution of an illness gives the sufferer 'special treatment and diminished moral responsibility'. Illness is therefore 'undesirable', a morally charged concept, whereas the concept of disease is completely devoid of value. According to Boorse "an illness is an affection only if it is sufficiently serious to be disabling, and thus (1) if it is undesirable to its carrier; (2) if it warrants special treatment; and (3) if it is a valid excuse for normally objectionable behaviour" [111].

Since Boorse proposed his theory in the 1970s, a plethora of objections have emerged. Boorse's definition of illness seems to lack an element that he includes in his definition of illness: the evaluative element. He is forced to rely so heavily on the rather shaky notion of natural function because he wants to avoid saying that what makes us classify conditions as illnesses is that they are generally bad things for the patient: this is one of the essential components of the notion of illness. To say that something is 'bad' implies that it has qualities which, all other things being equal, should be avoided or corrected: [112] a person who did not know this would not understand the concept of disease.

In other words, are infertile people who do not wish to have children sick or somehow in a state of disorder? Are individuals who have rare mutations in a gene sequence, but who do not experience any effects of these mutations, considered to have a disease? [113] Are HIV carriers who show no symptoms of HIV/AIDS considered to have a disease? Boorse has repeatedly and comprehensively answered these objections [114, 115]. In any case, Boorse's theory is a concept better applied by, and more useful to, the pathologist than the clinician.

Like Boorse, Nordenfelt argues that the word 'disease' is simply an empirical statement that should not be taken as an assessment of the person's condition. But Nordenfelt's holistic theory of health is different in the way it deals with disease. Whereas Boorse works his way up from diseases defined in terms of biostatistical deviations, Nordenfelt argues that we should work in reverse by first recognizing the suffering and lived experience of disease, and then examining the underlying cause of that suffering to reveal the disease state [116].

Clouser, Culver and Gert propose a different account of illness, substituting the concept of 'malady' for that of 'disease'. According to these authors, "a person has a 'malady' if and only if he or she has a condition, other than a rational belief or desire, such that he or she suffers, or is exposed to an increased risk of suffering, from an ailment (death, disability, loss of freedom and opportunity or possibility, anhedonia) in the absence of a distinct and enduring cause" [117].

But how can we reasonably make an objective medical assessment? Rational people would agree that suffering, pain, injury, and death should be avoided. But who are these rational people, and how do we identify their values in a pluralistic world? Are certain diseases that predispose to self-harm, epileptic seizures, or hallucinations, but which are valued in some cultures for spiritual reasons, objectively bad? These people are, as we can see, close to normativism.

Why do we get sick? Evolutionary medical philosophy believes it will answer this question because, according to Nesse and Stearns, "it will transform the way patients and doctors view disease" [118]. Pierre-Olivier Méthot sought to define disease from a Darwinian perspective [119]. However, it is now recognized that this approach lacks clinical relevance [120], especially since it is based on a very dubious view of disease and relies on the naturalistic paralogism [121] that confuses a judgement of fact with a normative judgement; and it appeals to a very limited view of evolution based exclusively on natural selection, and more seriously, on anatural selection that focuses exclusively on genes.

(ii) **Normativism**

Normativism is a theory proposed by Joseph Margolis [122], Professor of Philosophy at Temple University, Philadelphia, which rejects the possibility of necessary and sufficient conditions for identifying diseases as such: the concepts of disease and health are influenced to some extent by subjective values, i.e., beliefs, preferences, and goals that individuals or communities might reasonably have to achieve their vision of a good life. A disease, for a normativist, is subjectively disapproved by society, culture, or individual preferences. Rather than appealing to objective or biological characteristics, such as dysfunction, disease means something that has compromised an individual's values, that is, some or all those things that contribute to a person's well-being. For example, Lawrie Rezneck argues that dysfunction is not necessary in the attribution of a disease. Furthermore, the search for biological causes of pathology presupposes a subjective judgement about what is considered pathological [123].

Normativist theorists cite historical examples to make a convincing case that our concept of disease is inextricably linked to social, political, and religious values. The diagnosis of drapetomania (the disease that caused slaves to run away) was an example of the links between medicine and politics that led to ridiculous nosological concepts [124].

Homosexuality is an example of the penetration of moral values into the scientific enterprise to categorize these behavioural anomalies as diseases: it was not until 1980 that the medicalization of homosexuality was officially rejected [125]. To this, naturalists respond that these historical examples simply represent errors. We now know that they were artefacts of a certain ideology or moment in medical history, as were Banti's syndrome, or arthritic, cancerous or hemorrhagic diatheses.

But how do we know? By the way, naturalist would here argue that the objective criteria necessary to define a disease were lacking and reflected bad science: without an objective concept of disease; how then would we know if we were wrong when we called something a disease?

Michel Foucault was a normativist who proposed a critical, historical, and philosophical theory of the use of medical diagnosis. He suggested that the medical enterprise was a form of social control to lock up people whose illness, or in the case of mental illness, 'unreason' made them useless to society [126].

Similarly, Thomas Szasz—who was Professor of Psychiatry at the State University of New York at Syracuse—repudiated in numerous publications the fundamental concept of his own profession: mental illness. Psychiatric disorders are fictions created either to marginalize eccentric behaviour or to exonerate criminal acts [127]. In a sense, Szasz is a naturalist, since the only legitimate mental illnesses are in fact diseases of the brain. In rejecting the conventional categories of psychiatry, he argues that they are subjective.

Another recent aspect of political emanation of the normativist position is the links between the pharmaceutical industry and biomedicine in expanding the scope of the disease concept. The expert groups responsible for creating or revising nosologies often have links to industry, and these links influence their decision to expand the criteria for diagnosing patients or to create new diseases that promise additional financial benefits. This phenomenon is known as *disease mongering* and has been the subject of research in health policy, ethics, and sociology, although the idea that some stakeholders approve and motivate the creation of diseases is not new [128–130]. Intentionally fabricated entities or over-diagnosed diseases could include mental illnesses such as depression, attention deficit disorder, premenstrual dysphoric disorder [131–133], or erectile dysfunction [134].

This distinction between naturalism and normativism is like that proposed by Rudolf Carnap between naturalism and constructivism [135]. John Searle [136] also has shown a certain ambiguity in the use of the term 'naturalism' about which the advocates of naturalism and normativism are not always very clear.

On the one hand, there is external realism, which asserts that the world exists independently of the representations we have of it. This is the thesis that reality is radically non-epistemic. External realism is neither an empirical thesis, nor a theory of truth, nor a theory of knowledge: it is an ontological theory. The intrinsic characteristics of reality exist independently of our representations, that is, of all our mental states, which are themselves intrinsic to reality. Diseases are then predicates of ontologically objective entities or types of entities, for a naturalist.

On the other hand, if the ontological approach is about entities or types of entities, the normative approach is about predicates of judgment. The concept of disease would then be about ontologically subjective.

Let us conclude with Wittgenstein: "*Philosophy must not in any way affect the actual use of language, so it can only describe it in the end. Nor can it have found it. For it leaves things as they are*" [137].

(iii) **Hybrid models**

Hybrid models try to take the best of both models, naturalistic and normativist [138].

For example, Jerome Wakefield, a psychiatrist, and professor at the New York School of Medicine, proposes one of the most important hybrid theories: the harmful dysfunction model [139].

There are two conditions that must be met for a condition to be considered a disease. First, there must be objective biological criteria for failure or dysfunction of an organ or body part [140]. Secondly, the dysfunction is expected to cause a particular social harm or damage [141].

The importance of a comprehensive, holistic view goes back to the classic work of George Engel [142] and his biopsychological model of disease. He sees illness as a biological reality, a dysfunction, which can only be and is fully recognized and treated if the wider context of the patient is considered. A myocardial infarction would then no longer be a mere dysfunction of the heart, but it would also be contextual and part of the patient's personality, external stressors, environmental aggressions, or the result of a significant personal loss. It is therefore not a concept of a natural species or a social construct, but rather something real that occurs in the rich context of human experience [143].

Arthur Caplan has argued that a middle ground between naturalism and normativism is both possible and already exists intuitively in the way medicine is practiced. Albinism or hirsutism may be biologically abnormal, but with relatively little dysfunction, so they cannot be considered diseases. Although there may be social prejudice, the biological abnormality causes only a mild and manageable impairment, although in some cultures being an albino carries a stigma that makes the condition abhorrent. For albinism to be considered a disease, it would have to be both an atypicality for the human species and a more than minimal dysfunction [144].

In fact, Kingma has shown that the interpretation of the naturalistic and normative approaches as being opposed to each other is a mistake, as they are perfectly compatible. Kingma draws on Ian Hacking's work on social constructivism to show how social constructivism can be used to provide a means of combining naturalistic and normativist analysis of disease. The normativist can insist that values play a role in explaining why we have the concepts of health and illness that we do. At the same time, the naturalist can insist that the categories we use reflect a natural structure that can be described in terms of values.

However, the work of sociologists and medical historians makes it clear that the boundaries of pathological disorder have shifted over time: the idea that there are relatively stable concepts of health or disease is therefore challenged.

We may conclude, first, that the opposition of naturalistic and value-based accounts is a false dichotomy. And second, that the concept of disease must be adapted to the role it plays in the health care context in which it is deployed [145]. Thirdly, diseases do not have an essence, but fall under what Wittgenstein called family resemblances, for what defines them is a quorum of characteristics.

4.6 Criteria of "Disease"

Let us try to identify some criteria of "disease":

1. The disease state or process produces present or potential harm.

This consists in *biological negativities*, such as all forms of physical or mental suffering, infections, deficiencies, disability, increased risk of mortality, which manifest a value-laden biological disadvantage, and are termed "pathological".

2. Disease can be linked to *specific causes*, events, or circumstances.

Cases of diseases are biological processes that have known or unknown, intrinsic, or extrinsic causes.

3. Most diseases are not natural types but represent *medical constructs* and have no independent existence. Yet individual cases of disease have manifestations and an objective, real and concrete existence; they are part of the furniture of the world, but the boundary that separates and isolates them from biological processes is not part of the world. They are natural events but not natural genera or species.
4. Diseases have *a natural history*: there is a set of structural changes, both macroscopic and microscopic, that follow uniformly and sequentially from the initial triggering or causal event.

Most diseases have a pattern of overlapping and changing processes, resulting in a full spectrum that presents in all degrees of severity—not a simple dichotomy between normal and abnormal features—and have variations that are continuous with normal features.

5. There is a set of clinical *symptoms* and *signs* (headache, chest pain, rapid pulse, shortness of breath) generally associated with the pathological alterations.
6. Diseases are based on a negative, medical, *value-laden convention* that leads to a *prudential duty*: their negativities require medical intervention to favorably modify the clinical course and outcome of the disease process. However, while the need for treatment is logically inherent in the concept of disease, a disease is not necessarily treatable or curable.
7. *Biomarkers*

Biomedical research in the genomic era has expanded beyond genes. Thinking about disease in terms of "gene for X" has gradually been replaced by thinking in terms of "biomarker for X". The term biomarker refers to a broad sub-category of medical signs, i.e., objective, and observable indications of the patient's medical condition. A biomarker is "any substance, structure or process that can be measured in the body or its products and influence or predict the incidence of an outcome or disease". An even broader definition considers not only the incidence and outcome of disease, but also the effects of treatments, interventions, and even unintended environmental exposure, for example to chemicals or nutrients.

In its report on the validity of biomarkers in environmental risk assessment, the WHO stated that a true definition of biomarkers includes "*almost any measure that reflects an interaction between a biological system and a hazard, which may be chemical, physical or biological. The measured response may be functional and physiological, biochemical at the cellular level, or a molecular interaction.*" Examples of biomarkers range from pulse and blood pressure to more complex laboratory tests on blood and other tissues, to basic chemical analyses.

4.7 Causal and Descriptive Diseases

The term 'disease' is vague, as it depends on the criteria one decides to use to separate pathology from physiology, and in any case, there is no clear dividing line between its applicability and non-applicability. There is a multiplicity of definitional criteria as well as a multiplicity of meanings for the use of the word, and there is no single, defined set of conditions governing its use. It is not surprising, therefore, that the question of who is ill and who is not rarely arises in hospital wards but is not properly applicable to populations where illnesses exist as a qualitative continuum.

However, Brian McMahon has identified two ways of classifying sick people: diseases can be interpreted in purely descriptive terms (manifestational entities), or in terms of their etiology (causal entities). Two types of criteria are used to categorize sick people.

1. *Manifestation criteria*: sick people are grouped according to similarity of symptoms, signs, changes in body or tissue chemistry, behaviour, prognosis, or a combination of these characteristics. Examples are fractures, diabetes mellitus, mental retardation, the common cold, schizophrenia, and breast cancer.

2. *Causal criteria*: Causal grouping depends on the similarity of individuals with respect to one or more experiences thought to be the cause of their disease. Examples of diseases identified by causal criteria are birth trauma, silicosis, lead poisoning, and diseases defined by their causal agent such as infectious diseases.

4.8 Classification of Diseases

A classification is a way of looking at the world at a given time, writes Norman Sartorius. The creation of groups into which sick people are classified gives rise first to a nomenclature or nosology that characterizes diseases, and then to a classification of these diseases into categories that appear or seek to have a biological relationship to each other. The process of creating a classification is often even more arbitrary than the one that led to the nomenclature. Nevertheless, agreement on a standard nosology and classification, however arbitrary, is essential for communication between doctors or nurses in the field.

Ian Hacking has pointed out the interactivity that applies to classifications, and the genders that can influence what is classified. Hacking writes: "*There is a dynamic interaction between the classifications developed by the social sciences and the individuals or behaviours that are classified. The application of a classification to individuals can affect them directly. It can also change them. Thus, the characteristics of the individual in each class may change. Our knowledge of these individuals must then be revised accordingly, and we may have to modify our own classifications*" [146].

In other words, we would be dealing with categories that trigger a change in what they refer to, so that the categories can then change.

Wittgenstein writes: "*How we group words into categories will depend on the purpose of the classification—and on our inclination. Think of the different views from which we can classify tools by categories of tools, or chess pieces by categories of pieces*" [147].

Just as we might group tools in different ways according to the purpose of the classification—we might, to suggest an example, group all tools that need sharpening, thus putting scissors in the same group as the lawnmower. Words are not, as Wittgenstein seems to suggest, to be regarded as being of necessarily distinct types because they are not essentially of the same type. There is no more justification for one type of essentialist view than for the other.

Like the process of defining disease entities, the classification process depends on the objectives of the classification.

The International Classification of Diseases (ICD) has been published since 1900 by various international organizations and is now the responsibility of the WHO. Most categories are based on the organ systems affected by the disease. For example III: Diseases of the blood, VI: Diseases of the nervous system, IX: Diseases of the circulatory system. These categories do not imply that the diseases in a category share common criteria, either manifest or experiential. Two categories I: Infections and Parasitic Diseases, and XX: External Causes of Morbidity and Mortality, appear to be based on mainly experiential criteria. Category II: Neoplasms, on the other hand, is based on a very hypothetical and tentative intuition that there is a common pathway for all of them.

However, the components of a given category are extremely heterogeneous, so much so that some of them refer to conditions or situations that one would hesitate to call a disease or health problem.

Unlike the creation of disease entities, the process of disease classification has little immediate relevance to the medical practitioner. Thus, ICD does not serve as a nosology, does not really serve the purpose of a classification, but can be used as a nosology to provide a numerical identifier to facilitate, for administrative or research purposes, the constitution of groups of individuals for whom the same or similar diagnosis has been made. However, the ICD, although used to code causes of death for national and international statistics, lacks the detail often needed for morbidity statistics. For this reason, the United States, Australia, and the United Kingdom have developed nosologies that are compatible with the ICD in its topographic headings, but which provide the necessary detail for clinical purposes.

4.9 Are Diseases Natural Kinds?

The above hardly makes the naturalistic approach defensible and illustrates what Wittgenstein saw as an example of the 'tyranny of concepts'. Diseases, in our world, are created, modified, divided, deleted, enlarged, reduced, and finally classified into provisional nosological entities, by medicine and/or medical research. But clinicians and researchers have never been particularly upset by the lack of a single, universally accepted definition of disease: indeed, they seem to get by just fine without one.

Articles published in a famous issue of the *Journal of the American Medical Association* (JAMA) in 2001 illustrate that the concept of disease is inherently elusive and ambiguous, and that the implications of classifying and labelling diseases go far beyond the typical patient-doctor interaction. Both the concepts of health and disease have a descriptive component as well as an evaluative component, i.e., an evaluative judgement about right and wrong: a healthy state is better than a diseased state, and a diseased state is somehow abnormal or dysfunctional. A reading of these four articles highlights the exile in which the debates in philosophy on the question of the nature of illness are situated [148].

The tree outside may still be there when I stop thinking about it. Calling something a "tree" makes the word "tree" the name of that kind of thing, but the objects in that category are not human inventions.

On the other hand, if we collectively dropped all references to money, coins would disappear. Coins must be a rather different type from tree. Examples of what may be called "natural kinds" (trees, molecules, dogs, stones, etc.) are in this respect different from "social kinds" (coins, priests, soldiers, diseases, pathological anatomy, etc.) because they have an existence independent of our gaze.

In the case of instances of natural types, our way of thinking, speaking, and acting must be pragmatically confronted with an independent, non-verbal reality. In the case of social types such as diseases, our discourse is not so adapted. Diseases are defined in terms of agreement, but the content of the agreement can itself only be defined by reference to the concept itself. The content and purpose of the agreement are defined in relation to each other.

For epidemiology, all currently recognized disease entities represent artificial categories created by man and constructed more for their utility than for their "naturalness" [149].

It is doctors who use the term "disease" daily, while philosophers use it only in writings that only other philosophers read.

The idea that to understand the meaning of a general term, one must find elements common to all or to many of its applications has undermined philosophical research; for it has led philosophy to reject as irrelevant the concrete cases, which alone could have helped it to understand the use of the general term. Wittgenstein therefore advocates proceeding here by considering how any claim or denial of knowledge is made, and that this can be done by enumerating instances of known things [150].

Informed clinicians are aware that diagnostic categories are only justified concepts based on whether they provide a useful framework for intellectually organizing and explaining the complexity of clinical experience, to make predictions about outcomes, and guide treatment decisions. However, once a diagnostic concept has come into use, it tends to become reified, and there is a tendency to assume that it is an entity. This is where the endless philosophical debates between normativists and naturalists begin.

Recall that John Margolis, observed that medicine is a curious discipline in some respects, for it is almost the only professional specialty that claims to be scientific and makes its judgement primarily in terms of prescriptive standards. It does not limit itself to descriptive and causal questions but provides diagnoses of defects, deficiencies, abnormalities, infections, dysfunctions, diseases, and disorders—in a word, of various deviations from what are considered normal and not just statistically prevalent patterns of human functioning. It claims to identify norms of health and disease through the application of its own scientific competence.

Wittgenstein suggested: "*Philosophy is content to place everything before us, without explaining or deducing anything.—Since everything is there, offered to view, there is nothing to explain. For what is in any way hidden does not interest us*" [151].

However, it seems that instead of simply accepting things as they are, philosophers become obsessed with the question and fall into what Wittgenstein says is a misplaced and endless desire for explanations or definitions, when in fact careful descriptions are all that is appropriate. This is a common philosophical and intellectual malady, the inability to realize that at some point one reaches the bedrock.

4.10 Is Ageing a Disease?

Margolis [152] and Rezneck [153] believe that if we could find a way to treat normal ageing, it would be appropriate to do so and therefore we would consider it a disease. This idea has become increasingly important in medical thinking and research [154].

Ageing is not a necessity. Aging of marmots slows down when they are in a low metabolic state when they hibernate for eight winter months, and this is probably true for all hibernating animals. Hibernation slows down the shortening of the protective telomeres at the ends of four chromosomes.

Embryos do an even better job of reversing ageing. How do older parents produce younger offspring? A developing embryo reverses ageing and looks younger than the fertilized egg from which it was born. In a new study, scientists describe evidence that supports this rejuvenation hypothesis. Mouse and human germ cells appear to reset their biological age in the early stages of embryo development. A period of rejuvenation that occurs after the embryo is attached to the uterus places the growing embryo at its youngest biological age, called "ground zero" [155].

In 1825, the British actuary Benjamin Gombert observed that as people reached old age, the risk of death reached a plateau. "*The limit of the possible length of life is a matter which will probably never be determined*," he wrote, "*even if it should exist*". Since then, other scientists around the world have discovered further evidence of accelerated death rates followed at a certain age by a plateau in mortality, not only in humans but also in rats, mice, shrimps, nematodes, fruit flies and beetles.

At Stanford Universitý in California, Tony Wyss-Coray, professor of neurology, has observed that ageing does not follow a linear rhythm, but seems to accelerate at key periods of life; he estimates, in a study published in the journal *Nature Medicine* [156], that this is marked by three stages, the first of which is at 34 years of age, the second occurring at 60 years of age and the third at 78 years of age.

In 2016, a particularly provocative study published in the prestigious research journal *Nature* [157] strongly suggested that the authors had found the limit to human lifespan. Jan Vijg, a geneticist at Albert Einstein College of Medicine, and two colleagues analyzed decades of mortality data from several countries and concluded that, although the highest reported age had not increased since then, it had stagnated at an average of 114.9 years. It seemed that the human lifespan had reached its limit.

Two years later, in 2018, the equally prestigious journal *Science* published a study that contradicted *Nature* [158]. Demographers Elisabetta Barbi of the University of Rome and Kenneth Wachter of the University of California at Berkeley, along with several colleagues, examined the survival trajectories of nearly 4000 Italians and concluded that, while the risk of death increased exponentially up to the age of 80, it then slowed down and finally reached a plateau. A person alive at 105 had about a 50% chance of living until the following year. The same was true at ages 106, 107, 108 and 109. Their results, the authors write, "*strongly suggest that longevity continues to increase over time and that a limit, if there is one, has not been reached.*"

The question of the limits of human life conceals a more fundamental conundrum: why do we grow old? As the eminent physicist Richard Feynman said in a lecture in 1964, "*There is nothing in biology that indicates the inevitability of death*".

In a study published in *Nature* in December 2020, David Sinclair, director of the Paul F. Glenn Center for Research on the Biology of Aging at Harvard Medical School, and colleagues partially restored the vision of middle-aged and sick mice by reprogramming their gene expression [159]. The researchers injected the mice's eyes with a benign virus carrying genes that return the mature cells to a more flexible, stem cell-like state, allowing their neurons to regenerate—an ability that mammals typically lose after infancy.

Simon Carding at the *Quadran Institute* of Norwich University in East Anglia transplanted fecal microbiota for young mice to older mice, which reversed signs of aging in the gut, brain, and eyes.

"*Aging is much more reversible than we thought,*" Sinclair said. "*Cells can clean themselves up, they can get rid of old proteins, they can rejuvenate, if you turn on the youth genes through this reset process.*"

There are many varieties of aging. Although some of the variations in health in older people are genetic in origin, the environments in which people live during childhood—or even during their fetal development—play a major role, combined with people's physical and social environments, including their homes, neighborhoods, and communities, as well as their personal characteristics, such as gender, ethnicity, or socio-economic status.

An anti-ageing gene discovered in a population of centenerians by Monica Cattaneo, a researcher of the MultiMedca Group in Milan and Paolo Madeddu from the University of Bristol, has been shown to rewind the heart's biological age by 10 years. This is still early-stage research but could one day provide a revolutionary way to treat people with heart failure and even stop the debilitating condition from developing in the first place.

Growing old is a complex web of similarities. It is futile to try to determine this community in the form of a single definition. Ageing, the use of the word ageing, refers to a plurality of family similarities.

It is often assumed that ageing has an evolutionary purpose. Most longevity researchers agree that ageing is not an adaptive trait shaped by natural selection. Rather, ageing is a by-product of the diminishing power of selection over the lifetime of an organism. Selection acts most strongly on the genes and traits that help living creatures survive adolescence and reproduce. Selective forces act on individuals and their genotypes, not on species. Therefore, ageing is only a by-product of selective forces aimed at increasing the chances of reproductive success in the life of an organism. As the British biologist Peter Medawar observed in the 1950s, harmful genetic mutations that are not expressed until late in life could accumulate from one generation to the next because selection is too weak to eliminate them, ultimately leading to ageing of the species.

4.11 You Can Create a Disease That Does Not Exist

It is true that it is possible to create a disease that is not a disease. For example, macrophage myofascitis (MFM) was described in several stages from 1993 onwards by Michelle Coquet, a neuropathologist in Bordeaux, based on the work of the Nerf-Muscle Group of the Department of Pathology at the Henri Mondor Hospital in Créteil, and the Study and Research Group on Acquired and Dysimmune Muscle Diseases (GERMMAD). International medical opinion was then moved, especially as this condition had only been observed in France.

The World Health Organization then summoned the French representatives who defended this hypothesis to Copenhagen. They were confronted with doctors responsible for the International Classification of Diseases (ICD-10), who found no reason to accept this hypothesis and rejected it.

The conclusion is clear: there is no reason to conclude that MFM is a disease.

Munchausen syndrome is a patient who chronically fabricates or induces a disease with the sole intention of assuming the role of a patient [160]. This factitious syndrome is generally characterized by the inability to realize and accept the discovery and evidence of their condition: it is characterized by the absence of acceptance, as well as by the pathological adoption of a social role, a sick role. These patients differ from malingerers in that, although their deceptions and simulations are conscious and voluntary, their behaviour is not motivated by obvious external incentives (e.g., economic gain). Patients initially and sometimes chronically become the responsibility of medical and surgical clinics.

4.12 The Philosophy of Medicine: Essentialism

The axiomatic approach to the philosophy of medicine sometimes has the effect of distancing it from medical reality.

For example, Maël Lemoine has written a brilliant article, very long and exhaustive, which seeks to define the concept of disease by conceptual analysis. He presents the major contributions of Boorse, Nordenfelt and Wakefield, each of whom offers a successful definition of health and/or disease. The arguments they use in their conceptual analysis consist mainly in presenting uncontroversial counterexamples to a definition of a term that should succeed in taking them into account. He then argues that the conceptual analysis can arrive at both a naturalistic and a normativist definition of health and illness. It is therefore impossible to distinguish between them by further application of conceptual analysis.

Lemoine proposes to reframe the naturalist/normativist debate on illness as a debate on the naturalization of illness. He proposes to focus on the naturalization of the concept of disease, so that 'disease' becomes a natural term with normative connotations.

However, the naturalization of the concept of disease in the form of a general theory of illness is a project, not an outcome. It has often been pointed out that medical science has made enormous progress without a general theory of disease. Lemoine responds that it does not follow that the production of such a theory would be useless, and he argues that it would provide the means to understand it even better than we do at present and provide a much more relevant concept of what disease is.

In sum, Lemoine initially thinks that it would be useful to naturalize the concept of 'disease'. But he does not tell us to what end. It is the health systems that uses, creates, abandons, divides, and decides on diseases. It is also the health system that groups them into various categories according to their use, and their clinical, administrative, legal, physio-pathological, or anatomo-pathological features. It is difficult to see, and Lemoine avoids specifying it, what conceptual analysis could add to moving targets like diseases.

4.13 Fragility of the Concept of Disease

For most non-medical people, the concept of 'disease' is essentialist: there are diseases, each causing a particular type of illness. Doctors do not give diseases a metaphysical reality: they do not exist in an indefinite sense, independent of diseased organisms. They may use the name of a disease with different defining characteristics: it may be a clinical syndrome, a specific anatomical change, a specific dysfunction, or various combinations of these. However, confusion arises because it seems necessary to recognize two levels of discourse, medical science and everyday clinical practice in which definitions need not be objective and are not mutually exclusive, though they may be quantifiable. The practical nature of medicine is not conducive to theorization. Sometimes doctors are aware of dealing with other subjects than diseases (e.g., childbirth and circumcision of children).

Traditionally, the concept of disease has arisen to explain the occurrence of suffering, actual or potential, and disability in the absence of any obvious injury [161]. But there are other difficulties. When it comes to some of the mental disorders described in the DSM 5, doctors accept much more heterogeneous characteristics, since personality disorders or psychoneurotic disorders are such that the conventions by which diseases are defined no longer apply: the definition is then reduced to the need for treatment [162].

Three philosophical approaches have been proposed that seek to capture the concept of 'illness'.

The first is *epistemic*, EBM, evidence-based medicine. It does not question the purpose of medicine. It should allow doctors to work within its rules.

The second is *patient-centered medicine* [163]. This approach is based on the centrality or importance of the patient in the delivery of health care. It is opposed to *disease-centered medicine*, in which clinicians, through "scientific examinations" of a patient's body, locate disease in a particular part of the body and then prescribe treatment, without concern for the patient as a "whole person". Patient-centered medicine, on the other hand, is not only interested in locating the diseased body part but does so in the context of the whole individual, to obtain a "global diagnosis", including the psychological dimensions of patients' illnesses.

The third is a *value-based practice*. This is a framework originally developed in the field of mental health, arguing that values are pervasive and powerful parameters influencing health, clinical practice, and research decisions, and that their impact is often underestimated. Although it shares starting points with other approaches to values, it suggests that our current approaches lead us to ignore some important manifestations of values, both at the general level, relevant in legal, policy and research contexts, and at the individual level, relevant in clinical practice. Drawing on ideas from philosophy, value-based practice greatly expands the range of phenomena that can be considered value-bearing. It suggests that one of the reasons why values are neglected is that they are assumed to be shared when they are not apparently in conflict. Value-based practice is an approach to supporting clinical decision-making, which provides practical skills and tools for identifying individual values and negotiating them based on the best available evidence [164].

4.14 Another Conceptual Analysis: The Language Quorum

Wittgenstein opposed the Socratic quest for definitions.

First, he transposes the Socratic questions from a metaphysical to a linguistic plane. The answer to the Socratic questions "What is X?" is not given by the inspection of natures or essences—i.e., mental objects—but by the clarification of the meaning of X, which is determined by the rules of using X.

Secondly, he resists the idea that the questions "What is it?" can only be answered by providing conceptual analytical definitions.

In short: "*Don't ask for the meaning, ask for the use!*".

Thus, this approach offers a non-essentialist answer to the definition, revision, and extension of the term disease, which allows new characteristics, or traits, or attributes to be added to the set of those associated with the concept [165].

The family resemblance approach can be represented schematically using a symbolism proposed by Bambrough [166].

Assume that the "disease" has five characteristics:

I. A lesion in an organ of the body
II. It can be diagnosed by physical signs
III. It responds to medical treatment such as medication.
IV. It causes damage, such as pain or anxiety.
V. It is genetically predisposed

Five situations (denoted by the letters **A, B, C, D** and **E**) are then considered to fall under the concept of "disease". Each of the diseases has four of the characteristics, but each has a slightly different set of characteristics.

A I, II, III, IV
B I, II, III, V
C I, II, IV, V
D I, III, IV, V
E II, III, IV, V

There is nothing that these five diseases have in common. But they all draw, with each other, from the same pool of characteristics.

Let us now consider a sixth characteristic:

VI. Mental confusion

Does another condition F with the following characteristics also fall under the disease in question?

F III, IV, V, VI

F shares at least three characteristics with **D** and **F**. If, for these reasons, it is accepted that this is a new concept of the disease, another characteristic (VI) can now be considered as one of its features. It is necessary to judge whether the shared attributes count as a disease concept or not. This approach to the concept of disease reflects the fact that the meaning attributed to the similarities associated with the concepts is not given by the presence of similarities between the characteristics of the disease, nor by any pattern of necessity and sufficiency that these appear to exhibit.

Chapter 5
Mental Disorders

Canst thou not minister to a mind diseas'd,
Pluck from the memory a rooted sorrow,
Raze out the written troubles of the brain,
And with some sweet oblivious antidote
Cleanse the stuff'd bosom, of that perilous stuff
Which weighs upon the heart?

Shakespeare Macbeth 5.3.

Abstract Mental disorders pertain to the whole of an individual, a person, namely a 'self-interpreting animal'. Psychiatric classifications can influence what is classified: this is the loop effect.

Classifications of mental disorders are usually more useful than valid, and nosologies do not consist in mutually exclusive categories. Comorbidity be it accidental, etiological, or sequential increases in cases of mental disorders.

It may be characterized by fragmentation of the self, epistemic rupture, syntactic breakdown, semantic rupture, or a-rationality. Mental disorders may be the object of multiple realizations, so that supervenience is preferable to reductionism. Mental disorders such as schizophrenia may occasionally be adaptive. Wittgenstein views of solipsism proposes a new approach to the phenomenology of mental disorders.

Contrary to physical disorders, which pertain essentially to the patient's body, the concept of mental disorder concerns the patient's body as much as his relationship with the human and non-human environment.

Keywords Mental disorder · Fragmentation of the self · Epistemic rupture · Syntactic breakdown · Semantic rupture · A-rationality · Responsibility · Interactive types · Comorbidity · Multiple realizability · Validity & utility of psychiatric classifications · Brain bicameralism · Adaptivity of schizophrenia · Solipsism

A mental disorder may be identified by sequences of signs and symptoms, a clinical course, a pattern of distress and disability, a prognosis, an outcome, and an etiology. It may then have other correlates, such as familial aggregation, due to genetic or

L. Karhausen, *The Fragility of Philosophy of Medicine*, Philosophy and Medicine 147, https://doi.org/10.1007/978-3-031-41633-0_5

contextual factors, comorbidity, and a predictable range of outcomes following a variety of specific interventions.

Robins and Guze proposed in a classic publication five phases to establish the validity of psychiatric disorders [167].

First, *the phenomenology of the syndrome* in terms of cross-cutting symptoms: the presence of delusions and hallucinations characterizes a psychotic disorder, and the presence of a sad mood accompanied by changes in appetite, sleep, interest, and energy characterizes a depressive syndrome.

Secondly, *the course of the illness*: as Kraepelin pointed out, schizophrenia has a chronic worsening, which is not necessarily the case with affective illnesses.

Third, *family history* of illness or a genetic basis for a syndrome: patients with schizophrenia usually have a family history of schizophrenia or bipolar syndrome.

Fourthly, *biological markers* or laboratory tests can identify the underlying pathology of the disease; in psychiatry we have hardly any such markers or tests at present.

Today, we would add brain *imaging techniques* to study brain structures and functions, such as magnetic resonance imaging (MRI), functional MRI (fMRI), magnetic resonance spectroscopy (MRS), single photon emission computed tomography (SPECT) and positron emission tomography (PET).

None of these factors is sufficient to validate a syndrome. There is often a syndromic overlap, as in the case of schizoaffective disorder. Genetic data may be contradictory: patients with schizophrenia may have relatives with bipolar disorder. Treatment responses may also overlap antipsychotic agents may be effective in the manic phase of bipolar disorder.

Categorical typologies with their discrete entities are the traditional form of representation for medical diagnosis. However, dimensional models, with their quantitative variation and gradual transition from normality to pathology, avoid Procrustes's need to distort individual patients' symptoms to fit a pre-established prototype or stereotype, as they very often apply to sub-clinical conditions that constitute the bulk of patients seen in primary care [168].

"*Psychological disorders* [...] *I would define them as conditions that—not to question—lead a person to seek, or need, or be referred to the care of a psychiatrist*," writes Nobel laureate Peter Medawar.

Defining psychiatry as the branch of medicine that deals with the diagnosis and treatment of diseases of the mind is quite misleading. The definition of mental disorders used in ICD-10 and DSM-5 recognizes the existence of behavioural patterns associated with current distress and disability but avoids using the term 'mind'. They are diseases in the same way as non-psychiatric diseases: they are harmful processes, have causes, a natural history and involve medical intervention [169].

Wing and Sartorius observe that the term "disorder" "is used to imply the existence of a clinically recognizable set of symptoms or behaviours that, in most cases, are associated with distress and interference with function, always at the individual level and often at the group or societal level (but not only in the latter case)" ... "*Mental disorder is thus not intended to specify the presence of a disease, but to recognize the presence of the designated syndrome. It does, however, verify hypotheses about a pathology or other biological abnormality*" [170].

A major epidemiological survey found that up to 16% of the general population admitted to having experienced phenomena that clinicians would recognize as psychotic [171], and a recent study indicates that over 30% of the general population report having had experiences that can be described as psychotic [172].

Psychoanalysis was a major step in twentieth century psychiatry. Not only did Freud's contributions influence modern medicine and related sciences such as psychology, sociology, and criminology, but they were also reflected in the arts. Yet, since Jacob Conn's landmark 1974 article *The Decline of Psychoanalysis*, psychoanalysis has been gradually sidelined from academic psychiatry in most Western countries, except for France.

With Lacan and Kristeva, literature, with its wild proliferation of uncontrolled hypotheses, has competed with science and taken over the territories claimed by psychiatry. These procedures, according to Peter Medawar, are "*highly malevolent... for they represent a style of thinking that will impede the growth of our understanding of mental illness*".

Psychoanalysis is now the lost tribe of psychiatry [173].

5.1 The Mental Disorder

A mental disorder is a syndrome, and often a simple set of symptoms, and it has, in principle, all the common elements that define a disease, namely a clinically significant construct that is either a process or a lasting condition. To qualify as a mental disorder, a patient must have some of the following characteristics:

1. Mental disorders are recurrent, repeated, and identifiable patterns of mind disturbance, distress, and disability, actual or potentially harmful, that affect the whole creature, occur in groups, and are recognized by medical science; they may involve distress, mental suffering, excess mortality, and disabilities that impede the patient's well-being, achievement, growth, and fulfilment and make life difficult.
2. Mental disorders are also related to interpersonal disturbances, which affect an individual, a person or a sentient being as subject and object, as well as the relationship with his or her social environment, and which disturb the patient's relationship with others and the world around him or her.

Mental illness thus differs from physical illness in that its perimeter is not limited to the patient's body (as is usually the case in physical illness) but includes the patient's relationships with his or her unique environment and personal life history.

3. The concept of mental disorder presupposes the presence of a narrow range of causal factors, i.e., physical, or mental, operating within or outside the boundaries of the individual, which may be internal or external to the disease process.

Causal factors result from a plurality of underlying biological, i.e., presumably neurophysiological, and/or psychological abnormalities, and not from a simple mismatch between the patient and society. In some cases, a mental disorder may be a self-inflicted condition, such as an alcohol-induced disorder or drug addiction. Kant believed that mental illnesses take root within the patient's body, although antecedents in the social environment may play a role in triggering, maintaining, and ameliorating the process. Vulnerability to mental disorders is partly genetic and epigenetic, and likely to be influenced by the family or social environment [174].

4. Mental disorders imply health care need—not a demand—for prudential concern, help, advice, remedy, prevention, or care, which is embedded in the concept of mental illness, especially as patients are unable to adjust their behaviour or mental state by any direct choice.
5. Mental disorders, like physical illnesses, have a natural history over time.

Thus, the mental disorder as a process may manifest itself in a succession of well-defined stages [175].

A patient with a psychotic disorder may follow a progressive course with clinically recognizable phases.

(a) A premorbid phase with no obvious psychosocial impairment.
(b) An early prodromal syndrome, i.e., a phase of abnormal subjective experiences with transient feelings of depersonalization, self-perceived disturbances in thinking, concentration or attention, and initial psychosocial impairment.
(c) A late prodromal phase with attenuated psychotic symptoms (increased distrust, early sense of changed self) and brief intermittent psychotic episodes.
(d) An overt psychotic phase with full-blown psychotic symptoms that may progress to schizophrenia.

In sum, the natural history concept substitutes a scalar view for a categorical nosology of psychiatric illness.

However, some mental disorders are enduring conditions such as personality disorders and mental disabilities characterized by psychological infirmities and mental discomfort manifested by the presence of enduring traits that depict rigid and often stereotypical dispositions towards subjective experiences as well as overt behavioural or cognitive processes, and which may be exaggerations of normal personality traits.

Personality disorders—paranoid, dependent, narcissistic, avoidant, obsessive-compulsive, schizoaffective or antisocial personality are the most frequently treated disorders by psychiatrists, with an estimated prevalence of 10–13% in community surveys. They appear to have a genetic basis but may have their origins in childhood or adolescence [176].

6. Unlike non-psychiatric illnesses, mental disorders are characterized by the fact that the patient's attitude to his or her illness, his or her feeling or awareness of being ill, or the total absence of both, are an integral part of the disorder itself,

and are not something additional that can be easily corrected (as in pure somatic illnesses). Psychiatry is the only branch of medicine that necessarily uses a holistic view of a person, i.e., a "self-interpreting animal" [177].

5.2 Fragmentation of the Self [178]

What do we mean by "me", by the feeling of being "me"? The "I", as a private aspect of the personality, is meaningful, but it is not an entity: there is no need to try to discover it as an inner experience [179].

Ramachandran [180], director of the Center for Brain and Cognition and professor in the Department of Psychology and the Neuroscience Graduate Program at the University of California, San Diego, argues that there are four defining characteristics of the self that imply first-person awareness. First, we have a sense of continuity, of persistence in time, from present to future. Second, we have a sense of coherence, of unity, because we perceive ourselves as one person. Thirdly, we have a sense of embodiment, the awareness of being anchored in our body. The fourth is the sense of agency, of free will, the feeling of being in control of our destiny. Ramachandran's model does not consider a fifth component of the self: the ability to perceive and respond appropriately to the external world.

There are two prima facie possibilities for a break in the bundle, i.e., some break in the self.

Dissociative disorders consist of various symptoms such as amnesia (when certain areas of memory are separated or dissociated from consciousness), derealization (when the world and others seem unreal), depersonalization (the subjective experience of a disturbed self-image with a sense of unreality), confusion or alteration of identity, or any temporary divergent identity. There is an alteration in the patient's self-perception, or a dissolution of who they think they are, of what might be called their 'epistemological self'.

Conversely, *schizophrenics* may suffer from a loss of the ego boundary and have difficulty in experiencing the "I"—that is, who they are, their *ontological self*—and in accepting that their conscious and mental activities belong to them. They may lack an integrated reference system. Certain mental states, such as judgement or emotions, become fragmented, resulting in incoherent speech, and thought. What is divided or segmented is the inner unity of the self, the interconnection between emotional and cognitive states, with various fragments of personality co-existing simultaneously. There is thus a breakdown in the unity and continuity of mental states before and after the onset of symptoms. In this respect, there is a fracturing of the self [181].

Beyond this, Julian Jaynes raised the provocative question of whether the unitary self could be seen as an illusion created by Western cultural and social modes of perceiving reality, developed after Homeric times, and reinforced philosophically by Plato's account of mind-body dualism [182].

5.3 Epistemic Rupture

In everyday life, most mental dispositions have an intrinsic tendency to represent real or hypothetical states of affairs relating to the world or to themselves, which may be present or future, probable or improbable, desirable, or undesirable. Intentionality is that cognitive capacity to represent to ourselves our present and possible worlds; the attitudes or modes of presentation of intentionality such as our beliefs, thoughts, desires, wishes, fears, hopes, moods, perceptions, dreams, and the like, are 'of' or 'about' things.

A psychosis such as schizophrenia can therefore be seen as the realization of pathological epistemic processes. What characterizes misperceptions, delusions and hallucinations is that they are about objects that do not exist. They deceive their bearer because of the absence of a proper relation of the signs to the objects they describe whether the experience is taken as the perception of an external object. As a result, the mental illness is then a "*pathology of reality*": it consists of the destructuring process of mental states which precipitates the patient into the unreality of the imaginary, which will tend to be experienced and thought of as real for the patient [183].

Schizophrenics may experience an almost solipsistic tendency to focus their attention on their inner experiences, which deprives the content of experience of certain qualities of the mental or subjective while emphasizing the ego's sense of epistemological centrality [184].

Asperger's syndrome is characterized by a mismatch between cognitive and affective abilities. It can also involve a mismatch between a cognitive ability and a cognitive disability in the same person. However, for a person with extraordinary cognitive abilities, the diagnosis of Asperger's may be an intellectual gift.

5.4 Syntactic Breakdown: Deterioration in Coherent Thought, Perception, and Emotion

Psychotics experience a breakdown in the integrity and self-consistency of intentional processes, and the loss of coherence of these intentional processes can occur at a number of different levels that extend to the network of desires, motives, fear, actual decisions, and what links decisions to action: These disorders allow for a variety of mental difficulties, such as suffering from a diminished ability to engage in the social rituals of daily life, anhedonia or loss of feelings, bulimia or anorexia, attentional dysfunction, apathy and abulia, hallucinations and insertion of thoughts or any kind of inability to initiate and persist in activities [185].

Some schizophrenics, such as President Schreber described by Sigmund Freud, may manifest or even be aware of these contradictions and their paradoxical implications [186].

Rochester and Martin [187] examined the speech of schizophrenics by looking at what they called cohesive links, i.e., the links between sentences in speech. These patients use far fewer of these links and use weaker links that make it more difficult to follow the meaning of sentences: they use fewer reference links, and more lexical links, connecting words. Compared to manic or normal controls, schizophrenic patients show more syntactic errors and less fluency.

5.5 Semantic Rupture

If the relationship between the subject and the external world regulates mental states, a mental disorder can be recognized from any global breakdown or temporary or truncated impairment of the connection between mental states and the non-mental world, and of the ability to understand each other by empathic identification. In fact, if someone does not understand or misunderstands someone else's speech or behaviour because it is unintelligible, this does not in itself imply that the person is psychotic. Incomprehensibility is only conceptually linked to the attribution of insanity to the third person if the unintelligibility is public.

"*If lions could speak, we would not understand them*", wrote Wittgenstein. To which the cartoonist Peter Steiner added: "*On the Internet, no one knows that you are a dog*". It may well be that we cannot understand the lion, because even if it could pronounce grammatically correct sentences, its way of understanding the word would probably be too radically different from ours [188]. Wittgenstein's remark underlines the incommensurability of our lives with the phenomenological world of other species and our consequent inability to imagine what it is like for a lion to be a lion or for a bat to be a bat.

We have and can have no access to the subjective experience of another sentient being [189]. Yet to point this out is to ask whether our position with respect to the lion is comparable to our position with respect to the incomprehensibility of a schizophrenic or delusional individual. A severe psychotic and we are strangers. But unlike Wittgenstein's lion, and since a patient shares the same language with us, his or her mental disorder may take the form of unintelligibility or lack of understanding of himself or herself; this renders him or her incapable of rational self-examination, with a consequent loosening of emotional or mood ties.

In Thomas Nagel's famous essay: "*What is it to be a bat?*" he pointed out that even if we knew everything there was to know about a bat, we still would not have the slightest notion of what it is to be a bat [190].

Wittgenstein writes that "*human beings ... agree on the language they use*," [191] and that sharing a language, "*is not an agreement of opinion but of forms of life*". It is only within the framework of a common implicit agreement, of a certain way of seeing things, that we understand each other. And it is within this same framework that the incomprehensibility of the psychotic is described.

The behaviour and verbalization of patients with severe mental illness may be incomprehensible, incoherent, or unpredictable and have no rational meaning for observers. Speech and language disorders include slippage, tangentiality, neologisms, breaks or interpolation in the train of thought, resulting in incoherent or irrelevant speech. Laing writes: "*For long periods one had that strange feeling, described by German clinicians, of being in the presence of another human being while feeling that there was no one there*". For Karl Jaspers, the quintessence of schizophrenia is its incomprehensibility [192].

5.6 A-Rationality

Hilary Putnam [193], one of the central figures in Western philosophy, has argued that rationality and reasonableness cannot be reduced to formal rules such as those of logic or mathematics. Rationality is a capacity that is not exactly determined by formal or general rules. Wittgenstein writes: "*Note well that reasons are not here propositions from which what is believed would logically follow. But this does not mean that we can say: Belief requires precisely less than knowledge.—For what is at issue is not an approximation of logical inference*" [194]. It is not defined by a set of rigid, ahistorical, algorithmic, standardized canons or principles by which premises or certain facts lead to conclusions. However, this does not mean that everything is permitted!

The notion of rationality resembles those of health, function, physiology, or normality, in that it might be a default state. "*The reasonable man does* ***not*** *have certain doubts*". Rationality is a privative term and irrationality, or a-rationality has a logical priority. Certainly, there is no strict line between perfect rationality and extreme non-rationality. It follows that rational actions must be defined in terms of a-rational or irrational actions [195].

We can all be incoherent, tired, believe foolish things, underperform, be depressed and act unreasonably, but in general these behaviours have reasons and can be explained to make them understandable and intelligible, and to make them appear rational. An angry person is temporarily completely irrational: sane human beings are responsible, which implies a minimum of rationality.

Irrational behaviour is scalar: one can be irrational, and severe psychotics are at one end of the continuum. There are therefore degrees of a-rationality, and it is not a one-dimensional concept. The frequency of the a-rational traits, their severity, duration, and the extent to which they impair the individual's ability to maintain interpersonal, family and work relationships define the severity of the illness [196].

Kant identified three types of absence of rationality, i.e. psychiatric a-rationality (*Aberwitz*): first, a person with a disturbed brain may manifest perceptions that have no basis in objective reality (hallucinations : *Verrückung*) and in which he dreams properly while awake; secondly, he may have delusions, namely disorders of the imagination and of the ability to appreciate, evaluate and judge these false perceptions (*Wahnsinn*); finally, there are thought disorders (*Gebrechen*) concerning general judgments (*Wahnwitz*), such as hypochondria, melancholy, depression (*Trübsinniger*). Furthermore, according to Kant, a patient suffering from psychiatric imbalance (Gestörtes Gemüth) believes that his illusions and false sensory perceptions are the truth, because he resists all arguments and refutations [197].

Despite this, the delusions of people with schizophrenia cannot be properly explained in terms of deficiencies or interruptions in formal reasoning: in fact, schizophrenics may be more logical than healthy volunteers [198]. In a case-control study, Owen, Cutting and David showed that some schizophrenics show an increase in theoretical rationality. Under conditions where common sense and logic are in conflict, people with schizophrenia often reason more logically than healthy individuals [199]. The authors suggest that this is because they are less good at common sense: they may have a bias towards theoretical reasoning over practical rationality. Schizophrenia is therefore a breakdown of practical reason rather than just cognitive theoretical rationality.

5.7 Responsibility and the Role of the Patient

The essence of illness, whether physical or mental, is powerlessness and victimization [200]. Such illness is therefore caused and suffered rather than decided.

But certainly, the distinctions between the objective and subjective position, between third person and first-person epistemic access, are made by pointing out that our ways of describing and discussing normal, everyday personal interactions are very different from the way we talk about abnormal reactions and their appeal to a causal explanation. When we are confronted with a deviation in interpersonal relationships, we either talk about reasons and responsibility in intentional or motivational terms, or we abandon it altogether and talk exclusively in terms of causes. Both approaches can address many of our psychological traits, although not everything that is explicable by the first position can be explained by the second and vice versa. We therefore need both logical arguments for a full account of interactive transactions. In saying this, mental illness is the paradigm of those appropriate conditions of exemption by which one is temporarily or permanent.

On the one hand, in the case of physical illness, the role of the sick person is extrinsic since it is external to the process of illness. It is a social fact concerning a certain condition of an individual.

On the other hand, and in a certain sense, the sick role penetrates mental disorders. Psychiatric illnesses are illnesses of the mind, and the interconnection with the social world is part of the mind, and thus part of its disorders. It follows that the sick role is then an intrinsic characteristic insofar as it is constitutive of a mental disorder. Siegler and Osmond distinguish between the sick role and what they call the psychic role. "The sick role, they write, deals with what one 'has'; the psychic role with what one 'is'. They argue that this dichotomy is much more useful than the corresponding mind/body dichotomy because it substitutes a role choice for an ontological split [201].

Responsibility is a scalar concept in psychiatry. People under the influence of alcohol or certain drugs, people suffering from severe confusional or obsessive states, or some psychotic patients may be unable—and not only unwilling—to distinguish right from wrong and to assess appropriately the nature and consequences of the acts they commit. In this respect, Nagel subscribes to the idea that there is a continuum between the familiar interactive attitude and the objective critical viewpoint, just as there is a continuum between normal people and the seriously mentally ill [202].

5.8 Interactive Types and the Doctor-Patient Relationship

The important argument put forward by the Canadian philosopher Ian Hacking in a series of publications, opposed interactive types to indifferent types and defended the notion of a loop effect. Unlike indifferent types, interactive types—schizophrenia, infantile autism, or mental retardation are conditions whose instances are people who can become aware of being classified in a certain way. It follows that they may alter their behaviour, emotions, and self-concepts, which may consequently affect their status as instances of the type in question or affect its classification. Hacking writes: "*What was known about people of a certain type can become false because people have changed by virtue of how they have been classified, what they believe about themselves, or how they have been treated as such. That's the loop effect*" [203]. Classifications can influence what is classified.

It is one thing for the psychiatrist to adopt the objective attitude and to consider his patients as objects of knowledge. He examines the signs and symptoms and the co-existing biological, biomedical, psychological, and social characteristics. The suspension of his reactive attitudes calls for a causal explanation of why the person exhibits certain abnormal and unconventional behaviour. In saying this, what distinguishes the mentally ill is that they defuse our reactive attitudes and force us to adopt the objective attitude towards them. In such cases, just as if someone is morally incompetent, psychologically abnormal or under the influence of heavy alcohol consumption, we suspend our intersubjective way of acting, as well as our attitude of involvement and participation in interpersonal relations.

The scientific value of a theory does not depend on the mind of the scientist who develops or understands it but is based on verifiable objective facts. Psychiatrists are *externalists*: like biologists or physicists, they do not seem to be themselves part of the object of the exercise. Psychiatry—as well as medicine in general—is a kind of natural science covered by causal laws and, as such, is not supposed to affect the observed disorders. Wittgenstein says here: "*'Observing' does not produce what is observed*".

But it is another thing that the psychotherapist cannot escape a certain degree of involvement and participation in the interpersonal relationship. Certainly, the success of his enterprise presupposes that in treating his patient he establishes a kind of empathic understanding with him. A therapist must cross the barrier between the patient's external verbal self and his or her inner, subjective, and elusive world.

If, as scientists, psychiatrists are externalists, as therapists they are *internalists*, which allows them to have meaningful exchanges and to take the patient's perspective and narrative awareness of themselves. As internalists, their language is a performative and causal shaping force: their way of understanding the world is to change it [204]. The psychiatrist must question how people represent the world around them, including the patient and themselves. It is as if medical language is both outside the world when describing mental disorders and housed within the world through the therapeutic relationship.

In one of his literary essays, the poet Matthew Arnold (1822–1888) used the terms "*Hellenism*" and "*Hebraism*" to refer to contradictory elements of the human spirit. Hellenism values the intellectual side of human nature, while Hebraism values the moral side of human conduct [205]. Similarly, two psychiatrists, Philip Slavney and Paul McHugh, in the best (and shortest) volume on psychiatry one can read, have emphasized the polarity of Hebraism and Hellenism expressed in the contrast between viewing the patient as an individual and viewing the patient as a representative of the human type [206]. Two consequences follow from this analysis. "*Psychiatrists,*" write Slavney and McHugh, "*should know when to be Hebrews and when to be Greeks*".

This implies a real acceptance of what the patient is feeling. Dieter Wyss writes [207]: "*One should not underestimate the difficulty psychotherapy faces here, the need to find a balance between perceiving and being devoted, the need to see through the patient while accepting him warmly, the need to consider him not only as an object of transference but also as a full human being. The point of balance, it seems, is no sooner established than it is lost again*".

Furthermore, Rosenhan's study showed that whether a psychiatrist expects to see a distressed person, or a normal individual strongly affects diagnostic judgement. The diagnostic process can affect the diagnosis because it opens the loop. And anticipation can significantly alter the act of labelling a patient, thus closing the loop.

Charcot's assistants at the Salpêtrière Hospital artificially produced the symptoms of hysteria he described: they trained patients to act and prepared them each morning before the medical rounds in the wards [208]. "*Doctors need patients,*" writes Thomas Szasz. And the people who need help, who want help, are accepted in their role as patients and become a real occupant of the role of patient, thus coming full circle.

In our globalized world, several mental illnesses have spread like contagious epidemics: depression, hyperkinesia, chronic fatigue syndrome, post-traumatic stress disorder and various so-called functional disorders. This process of "disease spread" has been encouraged by multinational pharmaceutical companies, the media and health care systems, and is likely to place normal people in the "sick role".

5.9 Co-Morbidity of Mental Disorders

Comorbidity, which is the co-occurrence and not a complication of clinically independent conditions, is rarely discussed in the philosophical literature. It is usually due to *a common history*, but more rarely it may be *accidental*. However, a comorbid condition can also be *sequential*, i.e., a consequence of the initial disease. For example, cachexia is a multifactorial, multi-organ syndrome that is one of the main causes of morbidity and mortality in the advanced stages of chronic disease; it is a disease within a disease with metabolic and inflammatory features [209].

Physical illnesses, particularly chronic physical illnesses, increase the risk of depression. Some illnesses have physical changes that may underlie the development of depression, such as changes in allostatic load. *Allostasis* refers to the body's ability to adapt to stressful conditions. It is a dynamic and adaptive process. Tissue damage, degenerative diseases (such as arthritis) and life stresses increase the allostatic load and can induce inflammatory changes that produce substances such as bradykinin, prostaglandins, cytokines, and chemokines. These substances are involved in tissue repair and healing, but also act as irritants that lead to peripheral sensitization of sensory neurons, which in turn activate central pain pathways.

Furthermore, our knowledge of mental disorders refutes Cartesian dualism. Mental illnesses are not simply diseases of the mind. Wittgenstein wrote: "*...the problem of the two materials,* ***mind****, and* ***matter****, will dissolve... the whole world is made of one material*" [210] and "*Do I say something like, and the soul itself is simply something about the body? No. (I'm not that picky about categories)*".

A mental disorder can either result from or cause physical illness: depression often aggravates recurrent or chronic physical illness and increases the risk of diabetes, osteoporosis, alcoholism, and cardiovascular disease. Conversely, most physical illnesses have a psychological component: 50% of Alzheimer's and multiple sclerosis cases, 33% of diabetes, cancer and chronic kidney disease cases suffer from depression.

Patients suffering from major depression show inflammatory responses which are immunological responses to stress, and which are associated with autoimmune disorders. They produce more white blood cells, especially monocytes, and have high levels of a major inflammatory marker, C-reactive protein (CRP). Secondly, immunoglobulins can return and influence the brain. They cross the blood-brain barrier and perpetuate the depressive system by altering the functioning of the brain areas responsible for interpreting emotions. The result is a negative feedback loop in which inflammation makes the body believe it is under threat, produces a more robust immune response and perpetuates or exacerbates depressive symptoms [211].

As another example, a diet rich in fruit and vegetables, i.e., 'anti-inflammatory', is likely to have a beneficial impact on mental health, such as depression, and is associated with lower levels of perceived stress in older people [212].

In 1913, E. Kraepelin [213] wrote: "*Wherever we try to demarcate the boundary between mental health and disease, we find a neutral territory, in which the imperceptible transition from the realm of normal mental life to that of obvious disturbance takes place*".

Ian Hacking defined "biocircularity", the thesis that mental states influence and are influenced by physiological states. Hacking noted that "*changes in ideas can alter our physiological states*" [214].

But another question that arises today is whether mental disorders can blend. The prototypes described in textbooks are quite rare: atypicality is the statistical mode.

Most patients who meet the DSM-5 or ICD-10 criteria for any one mental disorder, themselves have criteria for at least two clinical disorders. This psychiatric comorbidity tends to blur the distinction between clinical categories.

For the DSM-IV, a patient who belonged to one category was, in principle, not representative of the other categories. But extensive comorbidity makes this principle rather fragile [215].

For example, 18% of the total population, or 60% of those with at least one disorder, have had two or more mental disorders in their lifetime. Or 50% of schizophrenia cases have at least one comorbid psychiatric disorder (such as substance abuse, obsessive-compulsive disorder, depressive or obsessive-compulsive disorder) or medical condition (e.g., heart disease, cardiovascular disease, osteoporosis, obesity, diabetes, autoimmune process) [216]. Comorbidity is therefore not limited to mental disorders: 20% of Medicare beneficiaries suffer from five or more chronic conditions [217].

The DSM-5 often includes a "*Not Otherwise Specified*" category, which reflects vague non-diagnostic conditions or those that do not appear to warrant a diagnosis. It is tempting to attribute the vagueness inherent in the concept of mental illness to our ignorance.

But this may well be in the nature of things. As a result, there is a growing interest in so-called subclinical disorders, since the disability and dysfunction associated with mild depression may exceed the disability associated with common medical conditions in primary care and the general population (DSM-5: #296.89; #296.80). Sir Aubrey Lewis argued that "*a gross psychosis may do less long-term damage than a simple neurotic: a dramatic attack of mania or melancholia, with delusions, losses, hallucinations, wild excitement and other alarms, may have much less effect on the course of a man's life than a deceptively mild affective illness that lasts so long as to become inveterate*" [218].

In short, comorbidity indicates either shared symptoms, shared risks, or the fact that one illness leads to another [219]. Our psychiatric nosography faces great challenges in accounting for the ubiquity of comorbidity, the inability of the categorical system to capture the full range of subclinical and atypical manifestations of a given disorder, the fact that distinct disorders can exist on a continuum without clear boundaries. The classifications overlap, and none of them is truly primary. It is up to us to choose the one that is provisionally most useful and has a decent predictive success.

5.10 Validity and Utility of Psychiatric Classifications

Assen Jablensky, Professor in the Department of Psychiatry at the University of Western Australia, who was Norman Sartorius' collaborator in organizing the *International Epidemiological Survey of Schizophrenia* in the 1960s, suggests that the prevalence of comorbidity undermines the credibility and conceptual basis of current classifications, as it tends to blur the distinction between clinical categories. The nature of psychiatric illnesses is such that they either tend to present in clusters or the diagnostic classification fails to distinguish spurious comorbidity from real comorbidity, confusing aspects of the same clinical entity with independent disorders.

Except for Alzheimer's disease, general paralysis, acute intermittent porphyria, Wernicke's encephalopathy, multiple sclerosis, hypothyroidism, vitamin deficiencies etc., current psychiatric nosologies do not consist of mutually exclusive categories. They are justified only by the fact that they provide a useful framework: for example, there is no conclusively defined disease called schizophrenia, which is a syndrome composed of a set of syndromes. Moreover, there is a continuity between normal and psychotic phenomena [220].

Jablensky advocates something like van Fraassen's *Constructive Empiricism* [221], a form of agnosticism about the validity of classifications. This position is a kind of pragmatism, and divides science into observational and theoretical statements. Bas Van Fraassen, professor of philosophy at San Francisco State University, considers that the latter are capable of being strictly true or false, but argues that the proper attitude is not to believe them, but only to accept them as empirically adequate [222].

Part of the problem is that the DSM-5 and ICD-10 adopt the term "disorder", which has no correspondence with the concepts of disease or syndrome in medical classification. This has two unfortunate consequences: the fallacy of reification, i.e., the tendency to consider disorders as entities, quasi-diseases, and the fragmentation of psychopathology into numerous disorders, many of which are merely symptoms. In contrast, syndromes are basic concepts for most clinicians. Jablensky suggests that these are good reasons to reinstate the term syndrome, instead of disorder, for a simpler delineation of current diagnostic categories.

Jablensky introduced an essential distinction between validity and utility in psychiatric classifications [223]. It is increasingly clear that mental disorders—even more than physical ones—merge into each other without a clear boundary between them, with overlapping genetic predispositions to schizophrenia and bipolar disorder as well as to the autism spectrum. It is equally likely that the same environmental or genetic factors may contribute to several different syndromes.

In other words, while most clinical psychiatric syndromes cannot be considered valid, many are pragmatically useful because of the information they convey about previous symptoms, outcome, response to treatment and, in some cases, etiology. Clinicians prefer and should for the time being stick to the categorical approach embodied in the current classifications such as ICD-10 and DSM-5.

5.11 Psychiatric Diseases or Syndromes

Raffaella Campaner, Professor of Philosophy of Science at the University of Bologna, in a brilliant essay entitled Varieties of Causal Explanation in Medical Contexts, constructs a nosology either of discrete disease categories (e.g., causal diseases) that remain the same despite changes in their attributes and clinical manifestations, or of continuous phenomena to which cut-off points can be applied to separate diseases from normal variations. The individual categories must be stable and distinct from each other and separated by natural boundaries: "*Medical science*," she writes, "*aims to identify the regular patterns of disease and to model them*" [224].

She illustrates the causal explanation of diseases, using the example of ADHD, certain pathways in the metabolic network, or certain rare genetic diseases. She attempts to construct some satisfactory causal explanatory pathways for such discrete entities, but she is not content with the identification of biological, psychological, or contextual processes: she assumes not only that a mechanistic approach and models are naturally suited to a multi-causal framework in terms of explanatory questions, but that they are also useful for defining and classifying mental disorders.

However, this approach raises more questions than it can answer.

Mental disorders are not mutually exclusive or exhaustive and can merge into each other without any valid boundaries separating them. There is often a common genetic predisposition to seemingly unrelated disorders.

The DSM-5 and ICD-11 are essentially classifications of diagnostic concepts, not of "natural kinds" [225]. The DSM-5 includes many disorders as well as isolated symptoms known in physical medicine as *medically unexplained symptoms* (MUS), or *medically explained symptoms* (MES) [226, 227].

A reductionist paradigm based on the molecular or systems level of neuroscience, such as that of K.S. Kendler, is a legitimate scientific approach, but it is clinically premature and philosophically highly speculative.

Certainly, a possible but unlikely scenario would be the advent of a "mindless" eliminativist psychiatry that is guided by mechanistic biological models and rejects psychopathology. However, it is far more likely that clinical psychiatry will retain psychopathology at its core [228].

5.12 A Note on Psychiatric Diagnosis

A patient suffering from a physical illness visits the doctor describing his complaints: swollen ankles, dyspnea, back pain, etc. In contrast, a mentally ill person never or hardly ever visits a psychiatrist: the general practitioner or the family refers him or her to a psychiatrist, i.e., the psychiatrist knows from the outset that it is a mental disorder.

The problem is that patients suffering from mental illness, as well as their families, are aware of the stigma and discrimination that comes with being recognized as mentally ill, which is not limited to the patient suffering from it but extends to the patient's family and to the institutions where treatment for mental illness is received, as well as to mental health staff in hospital wards of general practice.

General practitioners are reluctant to treat mental health problems in primary health care. First and foremost, this is due to their lack of competence because medical schools place little emphasis on training in psychiatric treatment for the GP. In addition, the stigma, and the myth of incurability of mental illnesses make the treatment of mental illnesses unattractive [229].

Psychopathological manifestations can be the object of multiple realizations. Different brain abnormalities may therefore correspond to the same mental disorder. This pluripotentiality rejects dysfunction as a criterion for defining the notion of disease.

5.13 The Fragility of Diagnosis

Mental disorders, like somatic diseases, are initially identified phenomenologically, i.e., by their signs and symptoms, natural history, prognosis, evolution and, exceptionally, by their etiology. Of course, rheumatoid arthritis or schizophrenia cannot be reduced to "what it is like to suffer from rheumatoid arthritis" or "what it is like to suffer from schizophrenia", but this phenomenological dimension, both subjective and objective, provides the initial material with which diseases, or at least the central prototypes of a disease category, are constructed and diagnosed.

The reliability of diagnosis in physical medicine is far from perfect, but it is much more valid than psychiatric diagnosis. In psychiatry, there is generally no specific physical data or biomarkers to support clinical judgement.

An exciting experiment [230] was conducted under the supervision of David L. Rosenhan, a former professor of law and psychology at Stanford University, who was co-author of one of the best books on psychopathology [231]. A group of perfectly normal people pretended to exhibit a single symptom, hallucinations, and managed to get themselves admitted to psychiatric hospitals; after admission they behaved normally and cooperatively. They went undetected and were discharged a few weeks later with a diagnosis of "schizophrenia in remission".

A second experiment was then conducted in which hospital staff were warned that at least one pseudo-patient would present within 3 months. The psychiatrists became much more conservative in their diagnosis. Of the 193 patients admitted, one doctor was firmly convinced that 41 were fakes, while another suspected 23. In fact, no pseudo-patients had presented themselves. So, what does Rosenhan's study mean?

Perception is certainly an active process. The meaning and value we attribute to a figure is partly provided by the context. "*A hand in the air,*" Rosenhan writes, "*does not have the same meaning depending on whether one is sitting in a classroom, turning right in a car, or participating in a German parade in the 1940s*".

In Rosenhan's experiment, the situation controls the diagnosis. For example, the fake patients spent much of their time taking copious notes on their observations. Almost a third of the real patients had detected that they were frauds and concluded that they were journalists or university professors. But the staff did not draw this conclusion. "Patients engage in writing behaviour" was the comment of the nursing staff on one patient. No one bothered to ask him what he was writing. But this apparently did not arouse any suspicion.

Once a person is identified as abnormal, their entire behaviour is coloured by this label. In Rosenhan's second study, each staff member was asked to rate each patient who asked to be admitted or who was already on the ward, using a scale indicating the likelihood that they were in fact a pseudo-patient. Doctors were cautiously more likely to label a healthy person as sick than a healthy person as sick. They were playing it safe, which is legitimate since it is more dangerous to misdiagnose illness than health.

Symptoms of mental illness are dispositional traits, i.e., dispositions to behave in certain ways in certain circumstances. But unlike other epistemic tasks such as science, diagnosis involves framing the relevant context: it is exercised within the boundaries of the clinical context. Friedrich Waisman observed [232]: "*No matter how hard we try, no concept is limited in such a way that there is no room for doubt. We introduce a concept and limit it in a certain direction; ... We tend to overlook the fact that there are always other directions in which the concept has not been defined. And if we did, we could easily imagine conditions that would require new limitations*".

A similar situation could arise if a false patient presented with a complaint of an intense and severe precordial crushing sensation radiating from the chest to the shoulders, neck, or left arm. Even with a normal ECG, such a patient would be admitted with a provisional diagnosis of myocardial infarction.

The hospital staff in Rosenhan's study did not consider the fact that people presenting to psychiatric hospitals could exceptionally be journalists pretending to be mad. Psychiatrists understand criminals may *pretend to be insane to avoid imprisonment, and they have developed* techniques to identify them. But they are not prepared to identify pseudo-patients.

There is, however, another important reason for the surprising results of this survey: the diagnosis of schizophrenia in the United States in the 1970s and 1980s was somewhat erratic, in contrast to the British standardized interviews, an error that has since been corrected.

5.14 Strawson and the Concept of Mental Illness

One of the leading analytical philosophers, Peter Frederik Strawson, proposed a rough division of the types of predicates attributed to persons in psychiatric grammar. *M-predicates* are those observed by a clinician, those applied to the patient's body. *P-predicates* include things like "is in pain", "is anxious" or "has an auditory hallucination", which are perceived by the patient. Strawson argues that there is not a first process of learning to attribute depression to someone else based on behavioural criteria, followed by a second process of attributing depression to oneself.

It is one thing to talk about a feeling of depression and quite another to talk about depressive behaviour [233]. It is tempting to say that feelings can be felt but not observed, and behaviour can be observed but not felt, and "therefore there must be room here to drive a logical wedge".

Strawson adds, "*We might say that for there to be a concept such as X's depression, the depression that X has, the concept must cover both what is felt, but not observed, by X and what can be observed, but not felt, by others than X (for all values of X*)". It follows that it is essential for the character of psychiatric diagnoses that they include both a first-person attribution because of the subject's statements, and a third-person attribution based on behavioural criteria.

Depression is not an object, not a thing, but a relatively permanent disposition to feel a certain way, which extends to first and third person relationships.

One might, with Wittgenstein, conclude that the kernel of truth of epistemic confidentiality is the authority of the first person: I am able to say what I feel, what I experience, what I think, not because I have infallible access to a private voyeurism, but because what I say, unlike what others say about me, is usually an admission, an expression or a manifestation without intrinsic foundation.

5.15 Suicide

A distinction must be made between suicidal ideation, suicide attempts and suicide. These are quite different phenomena from an epidemiological point of view, even though they are obviously linked: in 1 year, out of 100,000 people, an average of 4000 will have a suicidal thought, 180 will attempt suicide and 10 will commit suicide. There are on average 25 suicidal deaths per day in France; per year, there are about 200,000 suicide attempts and 90,000 hospitalizations for suicide.

Two epidemiological studies indicate that 93–94% of suicides had a known psychiatric disorder prior to their death [234].

While in 2016 the standardized rate of death by suicide in France was 22 per 100,000, it was 12 per 100,000 in the UK. In the UK, it was the leading cause of death for men aged 5–49, and for women aged 5–34. Suicide rates vary widely, from very high in Russia and Ukraine to low in Western Europe and low in Iceland and Finland.

A team of Welsh doctors has developed a new protocol, the Risk of Suicide Protocol (RsOP), to help health professionals assess suicide risk. In contrast to various previous attempts, this protocol now has evidence of its effectiveness in the form of two studies that demonstrate its efficacy as a predictive tool in both community and hospital settings. It contains 20 detailed clinical items that clinicians assess before deciding on the level of risk and determining an appropriate safety plan.

5.16 Mental Syndromes Are Realized in Multiple Ways

Psychopathological signs can be the object of multiple realizations [235]. Moreover, different brain abnormalities may therefore correspond to the same mental disorder. This pluripotentiality seems to allow the idea that mental disorders may not be numerically individualized since two people with the same brain condition may not have the same manifestations or the same semantic content.

An examination not of genes, but of the relative activity of genes expressed in samples of the cortex of patients with one of five mental disorders (autism spectrum disorder, alcoholism, schizophrenia, bipolar disorder, major depressive disorder), was compared with samples from patients without a diagnosis. This study did not find any similarities between alcoholism and the other four disorders, but bipolar disorder and depression showed significant similarities, as did bipolar disorder and autism spectrum disorder, and bipolar disorder and schizophrenia [236].

This leads to the rejection of the requirement that dysfunction is a criterion for defining the concept of disease. A disease can be mono-functional or multi-functional, so dysfunction cannot be a necessary feature of its definition, since multiple realizability would mean multiple functions, which would mean multiple diseases.

5.17 Supervenience and the Mind-Body Problem

Davidson writes: "*Mental characteristics are in some way dependent on, or supervenient to, physical characteristics. This supervenience may be taken to mean that there cannot be two events which are exactly alike in all physical respects but differ in some mental aspects, or that an object cannot change in some mental aspects without changing in some physical aspects*". For Donald Davidson's anomalous monism, every 'mental state' is a physiological state; but he denies the possibility of a psychophysical reduction of these states, arguing that laws that identify or otherwise relate types of mental states to types of physical states are impossible [237].

Naturalistic approaches to health and disease, usually associated with biomedical reductionism, present disease as a type of impairment of the body's normal biological function. In contrast, normativist approaches suggest that health and disease are value laden.

Given that there are a variety of different hypotheses to explain mental disorders and given the philosophical difficulties of the mind-body relationship, reductionism, for example that of Paul and Patricia Churchland, is difficult to apply in psychiatry.

In the same vein, Kandel [238] argued that the basic theory of psychiatry is molecular neurobiology, but this genetic reductionism, like Schaffner's, is a metaphysical and speculative position which Murphy [239] rejects for several reasons and which has not been adopted either in philosophy or in psychiatry [240].

On the other hand, supervenience is defined as follows: determining or fixing a person's physical properties (or possibly the person and his environment) determines or fixes his mental properties, but the reverse implication does not hold.

Holding supervenience to be true in psychiatry responds to the intuition that physical properties could be realized in more than one way. For example, in the case of computers, the same type of software state can be realized on different types of hardware state. The supervenience consists of a covariance thesis and a dependency thesis. This means that the thesis that the mind is supervenient on the physical amounts to the conjunction of the two claims: (1) the mind covaries with the physical, and (2) the mind depends on the physical [241].

The thesis says nothing about the type of dependency involved in mind-body supervenience. However, mind-body supervenience could be a special case of mereological dependence, i.e., the dependence of the properties of a whole on the properties and relations that characterize its own parts. According to this approach, we should explain psychological or psychopathological properties as macro-properties of a whole organism that covary appropriately with its micro-properties. The differences between supervenience and reduction are suggestive. The relation of supervenience is not, in the first place, a relation between theories, but rather between ontological domains. The idea of supervenience makes us recognize that the old model of reductionism missed the point by proposing a syntactic doctrine about the structure of theories, when what was needed was a semantic doctrine about the nature of the objects to which theories are applied.

Supervenience explains why fixing the mind does not fix the physical.

5.18 Can Mental Disorders Be Adaptive?

Although there is nothing globally good to say about mental disorders, when a patient's signs and symptoms are not too out of control a mental disorder can play a positive role in a patient's life. Psychiatrist Kay Redfield Jamison, who suffers from bipolar disorder, has provided evidence that suggests an etiological relationship between mania and artistic creativity, as exemplified by Coleridge, Byron, and many others. Many artists throughout history, such as Schuman, Dostoyevsky, or van Gogh, have identified with creativity associated with temporal lobe epilepsy and other neuropsychiatric disorders [242].

I believe, writes Sandison, "*that extreme and persistent depression is one of the states to which man is heir, and that its absence in a person is rare and more abnormal than his predisposition to depression*" [243]. The suffering of mental illness can be unspeakable, but it can also "*bring greater joy over long periods of time than any state of normality*". Didn't melancholy acquire a positive connotation in the 1600s as an affliction of people of superior intelligence? The mentally ill can also cope better than healthy individuals in certain harsh environments such as concentration camps or combat [244].

In addition, most of us tend to believe that fewer bad things will happen to us than to others. Most human beings are overly optimistic and tend to overestimate their potential and effectiveness and to believe that they have more control over circumstances and the way things happen than they do. Comparing the beliefs and inferences of depressed patients with those of normal people suggests that the attitudes of depressed individuals are often more realistic and rational than those of non-depressives, who exhibit more misjudgments and errors [245]. Depressive states may therefore have a selective advantage.

Laing, himself probably suffering from schizophrenia, wrote: "*Schizophrenia is a special strategy that a person invents to live in an unlivable situation*" [246].

Similarly, people with autism spectrum disorders may have better pitch recognition, superior visuospatial skills, greater attention to detail, and better rational decision making due to less sensitivity to emotional factors.

To summarize, mental disorders are not modules that can be removed from the realm of biological processes; nor are they clear-cut, distinct features that stand out from the context of people's mental lives, but are constituted from abnormal characteristics of maladaptive, positive, and negative traits [247].

5.19 Schizophrenia and the Darwinian Paradox

It has long been known that schizophrenia is associated with reduced fertility. Schizophrenia reduces the rate of offspring, so it is not adaptive in the sense of natural selection. If this is the case, then why is its incidence constant and uniform throughout the world (about 12 per 100,000 inhabitants per year) with a prevalence that varies between 0.5% and 1.5% in all populations?

The pilot study of schizophrenia led by Norman Sartorious and Assen Jablensky [248] has shown that the incidence of schizophrenia is the same in socio-cultural environments as different as a Taiwanese, Indian or Nigerian village and a large Scandinavian capital. The course of the disease and its prevalence, on the other hand, may vary according to the so-called "culture" and the context in which gene-environment interactions shape the clinical picture of the disease.

This consistent incidence suggests both that the disease dates to prehistoric times and that it may also provide some selective advantage [249] even though the formal description of schizophrenia was made in 1887 by Emile Kraepelin [250]. Furthermore, given that the frequency of fertility-diminishing disorder genes is expected to decrease, it remains an enigma how schizophrenia circumvents the effect of natural selection [251].

It is also conceivable that alleles conferring susceptibility to schizophrenia could be maintained in the population against negative selection by a high mutation rate. Furthermore, it has been shown that advanced paternal age is a risk factor because spermatogonia replicate much more during life than oocytes with a higher risk of mutation.

This may also be comparable to the genetic polymorphism comparable to sickle cell disease in areas with high malaria prevalence. It is sometimes speculated that parents, relatives, and siblings of people with schizophrenia, the heterozygotes, if not themselves psychotic, may have selective advantages in the cognitive and emotional system as well as increased innate resistance to certain infectious diseases [252]. However, the lack of evidence of increased fertility in relatives of schizophrenics weakens alternative explanations such as heterozygote advantage, and antagonistic pleiotropy (one allele may reduce fitness for one trait while increasing fitness for another trait).

5.20 Is Schizophrenia Adaptive?

There is a connection between schizophrenics and the marginal shamans of some primitive cultures [253]. There are no significant differences in the sequence of underlying psychological events that define their abnormal experiences. The main difference lies in the cultural acceptance of a life crisis.

On the one hand, shamans are men who communicate directly with their "spirits" in the other world and exhibit the most blatant form of psychotic behaviour, i.e., non-reality-oriented ideas, abnormal perceptual experiences, trance-like states of ecstasy, profound emotional upheavals, and bizarre behaviour. Prestige and faith in their power are generally given.

On the other hand, in the psychosocial environments of our Western culture, which do not provide reference guides for understanding this type of crisis of experience, an acute episode of schizophrenia has absolutely no cultural significance beyond proving its madness.

Sullivan concludes: "*The essential difference between the psychosocial environments of the schizophrenic and the shaman is the pervasiveness of the anxiety that complicates the lives of both. The emotional supports and collective ways of solving the fundamental problems of life available to the shaman greatly ease the tension of an otherwise excruciatingly painful existence. Such supports are too often unavailable to the schizophrenic in our culture*".

Entire communities—for example the Tanala of Madagascar and the Mohaves, a Native American people from the Colorado River in the southwestern United States—are known to live in what could be psychiatrically described as altered states of consciousness. They dream of supernatural experiences that are often confused with everyday activities, so that these communities could be tentatively described as psychotic [254]. A Mohave who comes of age must consume samples of Datura stramonium, a powerful hallucinogen, in a rite of passage to enter a new state of consciousness.

There is another consideration, which Daniel Dennett, a professor of philosophy at Tufts University, considers important. Julian Jaynes [255], a psychologist at Princeton University, became famous with a single book. Julian Jaynes and more recently, in a masterful book, Iain McGilchrist [256], have argued that the genetic change that led to schizophrenia and other serious mental illnesses, such as bipolar syndrome, was a necessary condition for the development of civilization and the reason we became human. It was this genetic change that was associated with the development of higher human consciousness and self-knowledge and that led to the explosive flowering of symbolic thought and activity, the arts and religion some 3000 years ago. And it is this same genetic change that has brought about the dark side of humanity, the agony of mental illness but also the nemesis of paranoid dictators. Much of the discussion is fascinating but somewhat speculative.

Beyond that, Jaynes' main point was that our modern form of consciousness and the suppression of hallucinatory experiences dates back no further than 3000 years but can be dated to after 2000–1000 BC when the mental solidarity between gods and people gradually dissolved.

In the past—and this could apply to the Neanderthal man who died out about 40,000 years ago—human mental function was characterized by auditory and visual hallucinations, in which people heard the voices of deities speaking to them and telling them what to do. The hallucinated voices reflected the activity of the right hemisphere, channeled through the cerebral commissures to the left hemisphere where language is dominant, and interpreted as linguistic statements. Schizophrenics indeed show a decrease in the lateralization of language. Modern consciousness only began when this psychological process was internalized and recognized as originating in the observer's mind.

But before that, human minds were split in two, the bicameral mind, resulting from a dissociation between the two hemispheres of the brain. Jaynes found strong evidence for this in Homer's Iliad, where the poet's heroes continually receive instructions and advice from the various gods. According to Jaynes, this is not just figurative language, but an authentic description of how people perceived the world around them. Beyond that, the characters in the Iliad lack insight, introspection, and self-reflection, lack our soliloquy and inner stream of consciousness. Instead, their resolutions, plans and inventiveness evolve at an unconscious level and are then disclosed to them by a voice or the ghostly figure of a friend or God. These voices are comparable to those of a modern-day schizophrenic. The difference is that they were not taken as something abnormal, but as a command from the gods. Jaynes described the same process at work in the art and literature of the Mesopotamian and Hebrew civilizations. Tethys came to Achilles and Yahweh to Moses. The first serious indications of the collapse of the bicameral mind came in the Middle Kingdom period of Egypt, around 1700 BC.

Jaynes did not equate schizophrenia with bicameralism but explored the parallel between the bicameral mind and schizophrenia. Hypnosis and schizophrenia, according to Jaynes, are a return to bicameralism. He writes: "*volition came as a voice that was of the nature of a neurological order, in which order and action were not separate, in which to hear was to obey. This ancient control structure manifests itself in schizophrenic hallucinations when the patient is invaded by admonitory voices that issue condemnatory judgements and command behaviour, just as it did three thousand years ago when men had no conscience and automatically obeyed the voices of deities*".

5.21 Wittgenstein and the Concept of Psychosis

"*I am sitting,*" writes Wittgenstein, "*with a philosopher in the garden he keeps repeating 'I know it's a tree', pointing to a tree near us. Someone else comes along and hears this, and I say, "This guy is not crazy. We're just doing philosophy*".

Although Wittgenstein was not particularly interested in mental disorders, his philosophy played a major role in the development of the notions of schizophrenia and psychosis in both psychiatry and the philosophy of medicine [257].

Schizophrenia has traditionally been described as impossible to understand both because of the profoundly strange content of the delusions that are among its main crucial diagnostic symptoms and because of the inconsistent epistemic and practical behaviour of patients. In 1913, the psychiatrist and philosopher Karl Jaspers had declared that many symptoms of mental illness (and delusions) were "incomprehensible" and therefore hardly worth considering except as signs of some other underlying primary disorder. Then, in 1956, Gregory Bateson and his colleagues, Donald Jackson, and Jay Haley, formulated a theory of schizophrenia as arising from double-bind situations in which a person receives different or contradictory messages. Laing put forward a similar explanation for psychosis as early as 1959: the strange behaviour and seemingly confused speech of people experiencing a psychotic episode was ultimately understandable as an attempt to communicate worries and concerns.

In saying this, a new approach surfaced in an academic debate between two philosophers on the following question: what light Wittgenstein's philosophy can shed on the most elusive, the strangest and the most philosophically charged of the 'mental illnesses': schizophrenia.

On the one hand Louis A. Sass [258] famously commented on the memoirs of Daniel Schreber, a legendary schizophrenic and author of a notorious autobiography. Sass observes that while somewhat milder deviations or insufficiently severe cases are, to a large extent, understandable, it seems strange to speak as if somehow there is some absolute line beyond which all understanding wavers, beyond which all interpretation can only be complete madness or total projection.

Wittgenstein comments: "*One of the main sources of our inability to understand is that we do not have a synoptic view (**übersichtliche Darstellung**) of the use of our words. Our grammar lacks synoptic character. A synoptic representation produces* *precisely that understanding which consists in "seeing the connections"*. Hence the importance of finding and inventing intermediate cases [259].

Wittgensteinian approaches develop a concept of delusion as a disruption of the enactive and intersubjective constitution of a shared reality. The alteration of experience is a subjectivity of perception, which results in a global experience of egocentrism and derealization. The delusion then converts the perceptual disturbance into a reframing of the perceived world, namely an alleged persecution by ordinary enemies. Through this, a new construction of meaning is established, but in a way that is fundamentally decoupled from the world ordinarily shared with others [260].

Thus Louis Sass, professor of psychology at Rutgers University and a leading exegete of Wittgenstein, considers that the word 'delusion', if applied to many cases of schizophrenia, has a quite different grammar from that of 'error': delusions are no longer mere cognitive errors, since they are not univocally believed, but form an alternative delusional system to that of everyday life [261].

Consider, he tells us, the sequence of Wittgenstein's notes:

> *The greatest happiness for a human being is love. If you say of the schizophrenic: he does not love, he cannot love, he refuses to love, what is the difference?*
>
> *"He refuses to love" means it is in his power. And* **who** *wants to say that?*
>
> *Well, what do we say, "it is in his power"?—We say it in cases where we want to make a distinction. I can lift that weight, but I won't lift* ***it****; I can't lift that weight.* [262]

The diary of a schizophrenic published in 1950 by the Swiss psychoanalyst M.A. Sechehaye, was written by a young patient diagnosed with schizophrenia. Perhaps one of the most remarkable passages in Renée's autobiography is the one in which she describes a transformation of the perceptual world in which the functional meanings of objects seem to disappear. "*Objects,*" she writes, "*are stage props, placed here and there, geometric cubes without meaning*" [263]. Such passages capture a perceptual transformation that many individuals with schizophrenia may experience but are unable to describe with much precision.

Moreover, Sass' main claim is as follows:

> *Schreber's mode of experience is strikingly reminiscent of the philosophical doctrine of solipsism, according to which the whole of reality, including the external world and other people, is but a representation appearing to a single individual self, namely the self of the philosopher who defends this doctrine. Many details, all the complexity and contradictions of Schreber's delusional world can be understood in the light of solipsism.* [264]

Solipsism is defined as the position that the self is the only thing one can know or, more extremely, that one's own mind, i.e. one's inner self, is the only thing that exists in the universe. This does not mean that one is the only human being, or mind, that exists, but that all that exists can only be either oneself (conceived as a mind or subject of experience) or a part of oneself (the content of one's mind).

Louis Sass thinks that the "*analogies with solipsism suggest that schizophrenia may be less a Dionysian disease than an Apollonian, or perhaps even Socratic, disease: a matter of the perverse triumph of the mind over the body, the emotions and the external world*" [265].

During his argument, however, Rupert Read raises particular difficulties for the project of interpreting people with schizophrenia, difficulties based on the apparent impossibility of a (self-)description of these people. The utterances of schizophrenics are usually interpreted as mere word salad, and it seems that any apparent order is completely illusory [266].

A profound psychic disturbance may deprive the sufferer of the resources necessary to enable us to make the usual distinctions in our social-psychological interactions with each other. Our conceptual faculties reach a limit, a limit of meaning, but not because of a poverty of concepts on our part, nor even on the part of the sufferer. We are not dealing with a situation like that of understanding an animal, but we are dealing with a system of non-clarity. The task of understanding cannot be "completed" because there is nothing that can be considered completed; even a limited understanding is of much the same sort as the understanding of a nonsensical poem that runs up against a hermeneutical limit that cannot be overcome [267].

There can be no successful interpretation of severe schizophrenia because there can be no true self-understanding of people with schizophrenia. No interpretation will succeed in effectively presenting the central aspects of the phenomenon, which are best regarded as senseless, as literally incomprehensible. According to current concepts of representation, delirium is seen as the result of faulty information processing or incorrect inference of external reality.

That said, any understanding, according to Wittgenstein, will be profoundly difficult, to say the least: how do we understand someone who is unable, as we have seen, to distinguish between 'does not', 'cannot' and 'refuses to', distinctions on which we rely as resources and as routine? How do we understand the world of a person not subject to these basic distinctions? Do we even recognize it as a world? The world of the unhappy and the world of the happy are very different, but they are at least two worlds.

Commenting on Sass, Rupert Read noted that solipsism as characterized by Wittgenstein in the *Tractatus* and *Philosophical Investigations* is impossible to describe, and incoherent as a concept:

> *There is nothing by which solipsism can be understood. The very idea of solipsism is ultimately a delusion of meaning. One can think of understanding it, one can think of having a clear idea of what it means to think that "only I exist". Wittgenstein's great achievement, in the wonderful therapeutic details of his later work, was to show that we don't have a clear understanding of all this; or rather, to show that there is no "it" here.* [268]

It is a mistake, as his opponent does, to accept a solipsistic interpretation of schizophrenia.

Moreover, he added, Wittgenstein's account of 'solipsism' regards 'solipsism' as a temptation, not a philosophical position or state of mind. In short, 'solipsism' is a tempting web of nonsense and nothing more, in which case it cannot be interpreted without violence into something understandable.

Schopenhauer, who influenced Wittgenstein, wrote: "*Theoretical egoism (solipsism) is only to be found in a madhouse and is not so much in need of refutation as of treatment*" [269].

It is significant that the schizophrenic type of world corresponds so closely to the description of solipsism—the illusory doctrine which, for Wittgenstein, is the quintessential example of the philosophical disease, that tendency to overvalue and reify abstract and contemplative thought and to lose touch with the true sources of wisdom that lie in a life of engagement and activity. According to Wittgenstein, this is a disease of hyper-thinking and hyper-reflexivity in which the coherent solipsist moves seamlessly from the idea that he is the center of everything to the idea that he is nothing at all; that is, he relies on the pragmatic absurdity of the idea that he requires the existence of another mind, returning again and again to a merry-go-round of philosophical positions.

Wittgenstein writes: "*'I' does not denote a person; "here" does not denote a place; "this" is not a name. But these words are related to names*" [270]. In other words, "I" can be a subject or an object. Or: "*In any case, I have only this.—What are these words for? They are useless.—Can't we just as well say: "There is no question here of a 'seeing', nor consequently of a 'having',—nor of a subject, nor consequently of an I"? Could I not ask: What you speak of and say that you alone have it,—to what extent do you have it? Do you possess it? You don't even see it. Shouldn't you say that nobody has it? And this too is clear: if you logically exclude that other people have something, it loses its meaning to say that you have it*" [271].

Wittgenstein pursues this point by considering what he calls the grammar of words such as 'here', 'I' and 'this'—words that are central to the solipsist's vision, for without them he cannot express his dubious claim. These words, known in linguistics as *indexicals*, tend to be seen as analogous to proper nouns, although they are in fact very different. In criticizing the dual understanding of indexicals, and in showing that the solipsist's sense of centrality, Wittgenstein knew that such a statement required a self-contradictory and impossible act, that of standing outside and objectifying the very structures of one's knowledge or speech. Such dualities and contradictions are strikingly like those identified in schizophrenia. These patients are likely to feel that they have unlimited power over events as well as the opposite and contradictory feeling that their actions, and especially their very thoughts, are under the surveillance and control of external forces.

Solipsism is thus, according to Wittgenstein, either empty or self-contradictory. Its central insight, the apparently bold and shocking assertion of the absolute epistemological centrality of the self either dissolves, reducing itself to the truism that what is experienced is what is experienced, or self-destructs, assuming its own contradiction. Yet Wittgenstein knew very well that the logical impossibility and incoherence of solipsism as a philosophical doctrine can hardly exclude its existence in the real world. He insisted that, despite their absurdity, sentences like 'the only reality is my present experience' correspond to a deep intuition of the centrality of the experience of the self to the world. Although this intuition cannot really be said (because it is absurd), it can somehow be shown.

In the philosophical debate between Rupert Read and Louis A. In the philosophical debate between Rupert Read and Louis A. Sass, it is the latter who seems to prevail, especially since the question has left the field of philosophy for that of psychiatry, and the Wittgensteinian approach has clinical and therapeutic consequences.

Let us add that Wittgenstein did not believe that the meanings of concepts could be reduced to a finite set of necessary and sufficient conditions. Even if there are rules of grammar (proper use of language) to be made explicit, these rules should not be rigidly applied. Thus, instead of trying to erase differences and achieve an artificial generality, the conceptual analysis should highlight differences where they have not been seen before [272]. Lilienfeld and Marino link Wittgenstein's notion of family resemblance to a special theory of diagnosis: rather than seeking the instantiation of concepts with rigid necessary and sufficient conditions of use, they approach mental disorders through the characteristics that lead to the choice of one category over another [273].

Elisabetta Lalumera suggests, in a very lucid essay, that Wittgenstein clarified the phenomenon of schizophrenia in at least three different ways: for the purpose of empathy, scientific explanation or philosophical clarification [274].

A philosopher and a psychiatrist from the University of Leuven, Van Duppen and Sips, in a study of a Wittgensteinian approach to psychosis, have shown that the delusional mood and the onset of psychosis involve the dismantling of the language game, the way of seeing things. The authors cannot distinguish a clear chronology or etiology and, therefore, find no argument to support one of the two-stage models of delirium formation that claims that perceptual disturbances generate cognitive disturbances or vice versa [275].

Language games and background beliefs constitute social reality, and they structure our perception of and interaction with others. Yet the habits we have learned from others and incorporated into our most personal ideas, beliefs and behaviours can suddenly lose their evidence in mental disorder. While the experiences of psychosis are often thought to be strange, bizarre, or incomprehensible, the aim of this article is to offer a new step towards a better understanding of how the psychotic process affects a pre-reflective background. The authors use concepts from Wittgenstein's philosophy to clarify the first-person perspective on psychosis. They describe the early psychotic process as a disruption of the "nest of propositions", shaking the scaffolding of our language games: "*What I hold fast to is not a proposition but a nest of propositions*", writes Wittgenstein [276].

Thus, the pre-reflective context that forms our existential orientation in the world is fundamentally altered. This psychopathological process transgresses the boundaries of language games, imposing a multiplicity of perspectives on reality, leading to the experience of groundlessness and blind spot biases. According to the authors, the perceptual, cognitive, pre-reflective and reflective aspects of psychosis are closely interwoven. Together these alterations lead to a radical reorientation of the experienced world.

Wittgenstein describes the flow of thought of the "philosophically perplexed man": "*The philosophically perplexed man sees a law in the way a word is used and, in trying to apply this law consistently, he comes across cases where it leads to paradoxical results. Very often, the discussion of such a conundrum proceeds as follows: First, the question is asked: "What is time?" This question gives the impression that what we want is a definition. We mistakenly think that a definition is what will remove the problem (like in some states of indigestion, we feel a kind of hunger that cannot be removed by eating). The question is then answered with a wrong definition, e.g. "Time is the movement of celestial bodies". The next step is to see that this definition is not satisfactory. But this only means that we are not using the word "time" as a synonym for "motion of celestial bodies". Now, by saying that the first definition is wrong, we are now tempted to think that it must be replaced by another, the right one*" [277].

Recognizing and exploring the depth and impact of this process on a person's world can be a first step towards resolving isolation and suffering. Philosophy can facilitate such an exploration, while interpersonal therapeutic activation can provide structure and confidence in the world, helping the patient to find a solid foundation in action and interaction.

The treatment of psychosis attends mainly to positive symptoms, such as hallucinations and delusions and repetitive movements that are hard to control, and therefore mostly forsakes possible negative previous symptoms that went beyond positive symptoms. "*The experience of groundlessness and blind spot prejudice is an essential aspect of the early psychotic process, which may remain long after the delusions have dissolved*". If, according to Wittgenstein, the foundation of our language games is an unfounded way of acting, and if we consider that the psychotic process is able to break the breeding ground of propositions that forms the language games, then therapy for psychosis should focus in particular on shared interpersonal activities—activities which Wittgenstein regards as unfounded "*but which, by their interpersonal character, can rebuild fundamental trust in others, in the world and in oneself, and thus offer at least a basis for recovery*" [278].

Van Duppen and Sips article combines a philosophical approach with a first-person perspective that illuminates aspects of psychosis that have not been described or elaborated before: psychosis involves an experience of existential groundlessness.

Chapter 6
Unexplained Physical Symptoms and Functional Disorders

It seems that the more intensive the investigation, the higher the prevalence of clinically serious but previously undiagnosed and untreated disorders.

Zola [279]

Abstract The incidence of medically unexplained symptoms (MUS) or conditions is over 50–80%. So-called functional disorders are unexplained sets of symptoms. Such people manifest illness behaviour in the absence of illness. As a result, the demand for medical care exceeds the need for medical care.

Keywords Medically unexplained symptoms (MUS) · Unexplained diseases · Illness behaviour · Need and demand for medical care · Disease mongering

It is often said that "medical science is about disease" [280], but this is a misconception. What concerns the doctor first are complaints, pain, and suffering, that is, abnormal and negative characteristics from which, by an inductive or abductive process, he makes a diagnosis that identifies one or more diseases, or is left with groups of unexplained symptoms.

If we could subtract from the world's population all the people to whom a disease is or could be attributed—assuming that all relevant medical information about them is available—we would be left with a considerable number of patients. People with diseases represent only a fraction, a subset of those with medically relevant problems.

The US National Center for Health Statistics (CDC) has reported that the incidence of "functional disorders", i.e., unexplained disorders, increased dramatically between 1920 and 1980 [281].

E. Shorter points out that the explanation for this phenomenon is not that people were less willing to take time off work in the 1920s, as morbidity rates for children under sixteen also increased by 233% over the same period. Shorter shows that the common diseases reported, which are the bread and butter of GPs, increased by a staggering amount: colds increased fourfold; sinusitis increased thirteenfold; urinary

L. Karhausen, *The Fragility of Philosophy of Medicine*, Philosophy and Medicine 147, https://doi.org/10.1007/978-3-031-41633-0_6

tract diseases doubled, and digestive tract diseases tripled; accidents and injuries quadrupled. The appearance and subsequent disappearance of diagnoses such as hysteria, hypnotic catalepsy, multiple personality disorders and neurasthenia were the result of changes in the way people converted their problems into somatic symptoms.

The symptom iceberg is becoming a major new socio-medical phenomenon, replacing the disease iceberg, which remains a central focus of health care providers. These symptom clusters are limited to the subjective feeling of being ill in the absence of any discernible and identifiable change in the function or structure of organ systems [282]. Shorter points out that patients, both men and women, show a general heightened sensitivity to bodily symptoms, regardless of their origin.

Somatic symptoms, not disease, are the main reason for more than half of all clinic visits. People complain of symptoms that can be disabling, such as exhaustion, fatigue, back pain, headaches, insomnia, rashes, pruritus, paresthesia, tingling, palpitations, restless legs syndrome (RLS), dizziness, weakness, breathing difficulties, runny nose, pain, insomnia, night-time apnea, or anything of the sort. These symptoms represent a major fraction of the population's medical problems and are an important if not major part of primary care. They may or may not be indicative of specific organ or system pathology.

The profile of symptoms observed by doctors is very different from that found in the epidemiology of the population. They are sometimes called *medically unexplained symptoms* (MUS), medically unexplained physical symptoms (MUPS) or *medically explained symptoms* (MES) when they last for more than a few weeks, but doctors cannot find a problem in the body that might be causing them [283, 284]. But the philosophy of medicine ignores them completely.

In sum, one of the characteristic features of the demand for health care after the Second World War is an increased tendency to translate vague sensory impressions that are not medically significant into illnesses, turning people with real suffering or existential difficulties into patients.

Our sensitivity to pain and discomfort seems to have increased over the decades in the Western world. It is not surprising, therefore, that our willingness to put up with them, our tendency to attribute them to a morbid disorder, and our readiness to seek medical attention have increased at the same time.

In sum, one of the characteristic features of the demand for health care after the Second World War is an increased tendency to translate vague sensory impressions that are not medically significant into illnesses, turning people with real suffering or existential difficulties into patients.

Our sensitivity to pain and discomfort seems to have increased over the decades in the Western world. It is not surprising, therefore, that our willingness to put up with them, our tendency to attribute them to a morbid disorder, and our readiness to seek medical attention have increased at the same time. "Diagnosis is the most common disease," wrote Karl Kraus.

In the Dunnell and Cartwright study [285], 91% of a sample of adults experienced one or more abnormal symptoms in the two weeks prior to the study. There is therefore a large pool of unreported symptoms in the community that are managed by self-treatment, with only 5–34% of symptoms resulting in a consultation with a primary care health professional [286].

Wadsworth et al. showed that 95% of a sample of 1000 adults had experienced symptoms in the 14 days prior to the interview, but only one in five had consulted a doctor [287].

More than half of the patients seen in primary care or population studies are medically unexplained (MUS & MES). Thus, people who experience a certain type of symptom, whether they seek treatment, may or may not have an identifiable disease.

6.1 Prevalence of Unexplained Clinical Disorders

Excluding respiratory infections and skin disorders, the incidence of unexplained conditions is over 50–70%.

Doctors and nurses are aware of the emergence of a mass of non-medical symptoms. Two hundred and forty-eight doctors surveyed in California thought, on average, that one in five patients had only trivial problems, with a consequent climate of resentment and mistrust when they find themselves overwhelmed by unimportant symptoms. "*They spend four years in medical school learning about diseases like renal amyloidosis and phenylketonuria. They spend two years in a family practice residency learning how to manage high blood pressure. Then they "treat" an endless process of colds, "treat" in quotes, of course, because a doctor can't do anything about a cold except let it run its course.*"

A Welsh doctor said, "*We doctors can't really treat the large proportion of conditions that come to us—they are not diseases at all*" [288]. After 20 years of practice in his own general practice, Dr John Fry wrote: "*The first shock and rude awakening for the doctor entering the field of primary care and practice is to be confronted with a mass of seemingly unrecognized, indefinable and unfamiliar disorders...*"... which "*cannot be neatly categorized, labelled or diagnosed with precision or on objective grounds*". This corresponds to the most noble and important area of primary care [289]. Several studies have shown that among 50–79% of all patients who present to a family doctor, no evidence of a specific organic diagnosis can be established [290].

Epidemiological surveys show that minor bodily symptoms are very common and that only a small fraction of them are reported to doctors: for example, a health care survey of the general population showed that 73–95% of community respondents had at least one symptom every 2–4 days. And 81% of healthy university students and hospital staff reported having at least one somatic symptom in a 3-day period [291].

These symptoms cause problems and are the main reason for clinic visits. They can also be subject to a process of self-amplification and self-appropriation: the more patients are convinced that their symptoms are abnormal or alarming, the more severe, prolonged, and incapacitating the symptoms become. Furthermore, the perception of bodily symptoms may be reinforced by stressful life events, or by becoming a patient: the role of patient may well become a way of life.

Nathalie Steinbrecher and colleagues studied the prevalence of medically unexplained symptoms between February and September 2008 in two primary care practices in Mainz, Germany. Medically unexplained symptoms accounted for two-thirds of all reported symptoms, with women, young people and non-native speakers having the highest rates [292]. There is a strong association between somatic symptoms and psychological distress. Anxiety and depressive symptoms show the same association with somatic symptoms, although some specific somatic symptoms or groups of symptoms do not show a differential association with anxiety or depression [293]. Some of these conditions are related to organic diseases that have not been diagnosed, but most are a series of coalescing physical and psychological symptoms with no evidence to support these symptom clusters. They may become epidemic and reflect a certain pattern of health beliefs prevalent at the time, but they do not fall into any category of organic or psychiatric disorders, and they represent conditions that we may be reluctant to acknowledge.

It is important here to exclude an earlier approach strongly influenced in the 1930s and 1940s by a psychodynamic interpretation of medical patients proposed by the Chicago Institute of Psychoanalysis, namely psychosomatic specificity [294].

It attempted to establish a certain psychological causality for physical disorders such as gastric ulcers, hypertension, asthma, or eczema. According to this model, particular types of unresolved conflicts produced permanent tensions and prolonged autonomic arousal, which in turn produced specific persistent or recurrent diseases. Psychosomatic specificity was compared to microbiological specificity since it was supposed to be possible to describe a personality profile or a certain expression or inadequate solution of an emotional conflict characteristic of specific psychosomatic disorders such as duodenal ulcer, asthma, ulcerative colitis, or high blood pressure.

Medicine was still under the spell of Descartes' dualism with a linear model of causality according to which psychological conflicts turn into somatic symptoms and functional disorders.

The DSM-5 uses the term somatic symptom and related disorder which corresponds to the ICD-10 somatoform disorder. Within this category there are several sub-classifications. Somatization disorder is characterized by chronic, multiple, recurrent, and frequently changing physical symptoms and a long and complicated history of contact with health care services, during which negative investigations or unsuccessful exploratory operations may have been conducted. This includes illness-related anxiety disorder, conversion disorder (functional neurological disorder) and other specified or unspecified symptoms and related disorders. Organic physical disease may be present, so the classification includes psychological factors affecting other medical conditions.

Marcia Angell responds: "*It is time to recognize that our belief in illness as a direct reflection of mental state is largely folkloric*" [295].

6.2 The Role of the Doctor-Patient Relationship

Although there may be several distinct ways of grouping clinical symptoms, it is the doctor who shapes the diagnostic label given to the patient. "*Could it be*," writes Allen Barbour, "*that we diagnose what we 'want' to diagnose*?" The same polysymptomatic clinical picture may be diagnosed as chronic fatigue syndrome by an internist, alexithymia or hypochondria by a psychiatrist, or fibromyalgia by a rheumatologist. Increasingly, expert consensus is used to legitimize groups of symptoms, which can then become entrenched [296].

Daniel Kahneman observes that if a doctor has seen two cases of a particular disease, he or she is likely to see more cases of that disease than someone who has not. Doctors may also have different ways of looking at cases, such as different orders in which they consider diagnoses. If a diagnosis comes more easily to the mind of one doctor than another, he or she is more likely to make that diagnosis.

The doctor-patient relationship is therefore particularly important in these conditions. Unmet expectations related to symptoms—including the desire for diagnostic and prognostic information—when met, can potentially alleviate symptoms, and reduce concerns about serious illness. And there is an association between multiple physical symptoms and the difficulty of the doctor-patient relationship that increases with the number of unexplained physical symptoms [297].

The diagnosis becomes a moving target with a loop effect, and functional disorders mutate in a complex cultural and biomedical context. And since symptoms and functional disorders are now the main clinical and public health problems, it is not surprising that the level of job satisfaction has decreased considerably in recent decades [298].

Physicians can foster patients' somatizing fixation and reinforce illness-related beliefs and behaviours: in fact, patients and physicians look for biomedical reasons, and are both concerned when diagnostic tests find no biomedical cause. The provision of medical care can trigger a self-perpetuating process of medicalization, a classificatory loop [299], which may well increase the severity of the patient's complaints [300]. Thus, doctors and patients become involved together in a kind of self-fulfilling prophecy through a feedback effect, in a vicious circle of unnecessary medical interventions and increasing frustration on both sides, which reinforce each other. Medical doctrine and lay opinion reflect and modify each other, so that what may appear to be a new disease does not reflect new knowledge, but a change in the character of an unstable condition due to changes in its representation [301].

The expression of symptoms may be reinforced by the amplification of normal body symptoms. This either allows the patient to escape and avoid anxiety-provoking situations, or to enter the role of the sick person when social comfort and medical care are provided. Symptom clusters develop when expected patterns and cultural stereotypes shape them. As an illustration, "normal" premenstrual physical and psychological changes trigger a process of misattribution conditioning due to women's learned expectations. Premenstrual changes are modelled on a medical or mental disorder, now called ‘dysphoric disorder’ or ‘premenstrual syndrome’: symptoms are modelled by other women as expected female role models and are then reinforced by medical care through Ian Hacking’s loop effect.

6.3 Cultural Factors and Disease as Behaviour

Plato wrote: “Surely there is no worse obstacle than that excessive care of the body beyond the exercise it needs to remain in good health... The constant apprehension of headaches and dizziness, for which study is held responsible, is an obstacle to any exercise or test of intellectual quality, when a man always imagines himself to be ill and never ceases to worry about his body.

“*Illness behaviour*,” a term introduced by Rutgers University professor David Mechanic, can be defined as the observable and potentially measurable actions and behaviours that express the individual’s differential perception and evaluation of medical symptoms and body signals. In fact, illness behaviour is not something that happens to someone, but something that they do: it is expressive rather than descriptive. The role of primary care is then to teach patients to pay less attention to their symptoms and not to read them as a harbinger of disaster, even if the symptoms do not go away. Thus, in a way, they are “real”. Patients form negative cognitive evaluations of their symptoms because they think that fatigue, pain, or discomfort are indicative of disease.

But this can become difficult to manage when the presentation of symptoms does not fit the social and cultural norms in question. In extreme cases, the attention paid to them is so disproportionate and disabling that the patient becomes absorbed in their symptoms, whether organic or not. When the reaction to symptoms is amplified, this creates an epistemic gap between the manifestations of the disease behaviour and its medical reality, or the disabling perception of normal body signals and their objective meaning. So-called functional disorders and symptom complexes result from an over-interpretation of normal body sensations.

It is therefore not surprising that the demand for care far exceeds the need for care. This leads to a high consumption of medical care with frequent hospitalizations and repeated surgeries. Tranquilizers are therefore increasingly used for cosmetic rather than therapeutic pharmacology. This is conducive to defining more and more life events as illnesses, and to expanding the scope of medical care.

In this respect, there is a dangerous tendency in public, political and medical opinion to regard everyday behavioural difficulties as medical problems. There is no doubt that pharmaceutical companies are reinforcing this trend, bending the will of politicians, doctors, and the public through a process of *disease mongering* that is damaging to individuals and health services. There is a growing stream of so-called cures for diseases that people never thought they had: testosterone for male aging syndrome, Ritalin for hyperkinetic children, or tranquilizers for existential problems.

It is also remarkable that these non-medical disorders appear and develop cultures, places, and ages, i.e., in a particular social and historical context. Take, for example, an epidemic disease that had a devastating impact on a high school in McMinnville, Tennessee. The symptoms attributed to exposure to toxic fumes had the characteristics of a psychogenic mass illness, including generalized subjective symptoms thought to be due to exposure to a toxic substance in the environment, in the absence of objective evidence of an environmental cause.

Electro hypersensitivity syndrome has little to do with electromagnetic radiation, since medical investigations have failed to demonstrate a causal relationship between exposure to electromagnetic radiation and EHS, a relationship that is highly unlikely for a physicist. It is a phobia of anxiety disorders reinforced by the media, which make people focus on mobile phones, antennas, or radio frequency transmitters: the media, which insist on a supposedly dangerous exposure, increase the probability of experiencing symptoms after a fictitious exposure.

Strong pressure from the demand side sometimes creates new needs. Public opinion and medical care can exert a causal influence, manipulate, and shape clinical categories and functional deviations. Dancing manias such as St. Vitus dancing and tarantism, lycanthropy in which people thought they were wolves, multiple personality syndrome, electromagnetic hypersensitivity, multiple chemical sensitivity, or Gulf War syndrome as well as the hysteria syndrome described by Charcot and Freud are manifestations of complex psychological artefacts, often created by the joint efforts of enthusiastic therapists and malleable patients. Excluding malingering, their victims are engaged in the staging of expected symptoms, which are involuntarily induced by suggestive questions.

In addition, there are many contextual factors that compound the problems. For example, the deep distrust of medical expertise and the consequent frequent use of alternative medicine, the effect of litigation and health insurance compensation, and the gathering of lobbies and pressure groups that push for acceptance of a functional entity that they turn into a subculture, such as the alleged carcinogenic risk of glyphosate. Eventually, patients take over and become active public advocates for these syndromes in the controversy over their legitimacy.

In 1893, Gowers (1845–1915) believed that a large proportion of patients suffered from "*diseases which consist only of a disturbance of function: ... they are transient and not permanent and are not known to depend on organic changes*" [302].

Societal and biological factors determine, so to speak, the role of the patient in our therapeutic culture, as well as, to some extent, the classification schemes and naming of these unexplained and unstructured conditions, in contrast to diseases whose names, classifications, causes and diagnostic criteria depend much less on cultural factors than on accumulated clinical and epidemiological data [303].

What characterizes these disorders is that, since they are largely socially constructed, unlike physical and mental illnesses, they are not inevitable and are constantly changing. Unlike paradigmatic illnesses, these symptom complexes are not disjointed sets: they meet the diagnostic criteria of several, often overlapping, conditions, and they change in response to technological, environmental, and cultural concerns. Illnesses that were traditionally considered to be moral are now medicalized [304].

But these symptom clusters have another distinct feature: while the need for intervention is constitutive of what is meant by 'illness', the intervention in this case is not a medical need, but a social demand. These patients have explicit and fixed beliefs and phobias about their condition. They tend to hold on to their "sick role" beliefs in the face of any effort to dislodge them. Their symptoms are generally difficult to alleviate and are not affected by reassurance, explanation, and symptomatic treatment.

Chronic fatigue syndrome (CFS), originally called myalgic encephalomyelitis (ME), is a disabling illness that often persists for months or years, accompanied by extreme weakness, inability to think straight, disturbed sleep and headaches, with no apparent link to demographic or psychological factors. Rather than being a specific disease, it may be the terminal phase of several diseases: infectious mononucleosis, influenza-like illnesses or COVID-19 have been shown to trigger this syndrome [305].

6.4 Conclusion

Functional disorders and unexplained symptoms are major manifestations that remain irreducible or isolated from conventional medical pathways. While the concept of disease dominates our medical thinking, functional disorders take the lion's share of primary medical care, constituting a large proportion of reported and unreported medical complaints, and causing absenteeism, lost productivity, and unnecessary medical costs. Many of these patients assume the role of sick without probably being sick. Unexplained symptoms or their clusters, whether reported or not, are not just diagnostic garbage: they may or may not require or justify medical care, but they reveal a specific demand and expectation for care.

"*Theoretical health is the absence of disease*", writes Boorse. But it should be clear by now that this view is wrong since many, if not most, disease processes encountered in the general population and in clinical medicine are not diseases. Once patients have been classified and fitted into the appropriate niches, there remain many individuals who complain of generic symptoms suggestive of physical disease, but who cannot be accurately categorized.

These people are not malingerers, as their complaints are real. These multifaceted disorders once again point to the responsibility of the press and television for their role in triggering and disseminating them, as well as for their reluctance or lack of critical thinking. It is therefore not surprising that public opinion has medicalized existential problems into putative diseases that have no chance of entering either the International Classification of Diseases (ICD-10) or any nosography.

Chapter 7
Health

> *A person can feel healthy and never know if he is healthy.*
> Kant

Abstract For WHO, health is a state of complete physical, mental, and social well-being and not merely the absence of disease or infirmity. However, it is possible to be sick and healthy at the same time. Health is a graded, scalar, measurable rather than dichotomous variable. There are many definitions, but no universal definition of health. There are different systems of rules corresponding to different language games that will appropriately be defined by usage.

Keywords Health · WHO · Social well-being · Homeostasis · Naturalism · Health as a graded continuum · Family resemblances

The concept of health is of a different nature from that of illness. Sick people can be observed and described in a doctor's surgery, or in a hospital or health center. They are countable and can be interviewed, examined, described, diagnostic tests and measurements can be carried out, and an attempt made to classify them into categories of disease. People with a disease, diabetes, typhoid fever, or hyperthyroidism, are therefore natural and objective phenomena.

On the other hand, it is difficult to identify, count and describe healthy people, because the concept of health is a subjective, global, contextual, evolving, and multidimensional qualification. If it were possible to describe a person as 'healthy', it would not be a natural phenomenon but a subjective judgement or a theoretical construct.

What mobilizes people is suffering, unmanageable disability and illness, i.e., ill health. When expectations are not met, there is a cry for help. When expectations are met, nothing is usually said. It is a matter of feeling rather than statistics; health is one of life's great blessings, yet we are not aware of it while we have it but become aware of it after we lose it.

What are the origins of the term 'health'.

L. Karhausen, *The Fragility of Philosophy of Medicine*, Philosophy and Medicine 147, https://doi.org/10.1007/978-3-031-41633-0_7

The Latin words "salus" and "malus" are transmitted into French as "salut" and "maladie". "Salus" means health, rescue, redemption and wealth and it derives from "salvus" which means safe, alive, healthy, unharmed.

In English, "health" derives from the Old English "hælth", which is related to "whole", "a thing that is complete in itself" (Oxford Dictionary), which in turn is derived from "hal" of Germanic origin, which relates health, fullness, happiness, and salvation.

7.1 The WHO Definition of Health

In 1948, WHO defined health as "a state of complete physical, mental and social well-being and not merely the absence of disease or infirmity". R.S. Downie believes that this definition is a step in the right direction. Health cannot be defined as the mere absence of disease or infirmity, especially as a person may have an illness without feeling ill, and may experience unwanted symptoms such as headaches, fainting or vomiting, when no disease is present. It may be the normal infirmity of old age or a kind of deformity, but the person with it is not necessarily in poor health.

While quality of life is often cited as central to definitions and theories of health, many commentators are wary of extending the WHO terminology, as it seems to encompass many things other than the health of the individual that might contribute to, or detract from, well-being. On the one hand, health is a pleasurable state, intrinsically and instrumentally valuable, and on the other, it has mental and social dimensions. It is its identification with human well-being, a notoriously ambiguous concept, that some critics have rejected. For example, D. Callahan [306] and Wylie [307] argue that the medicalization of social problems proposed by this definition might suggest that all social ills are caused by or exemplify ill health.

A narrower definition of health sees its legitimate domain as the state that medicine seeks to restore, and its opposite being 'ill health' rather than disease as such. Callahan observed that, intuitively, health is a medical norm and a moral ideal [308]. As a standard, it is a matter of the heart, lungs, kidneys, and other parts of the body functioning to a threshold of normality that can be established empirically and statistically.

A positive sense of well-being is not enough. According to Downie, "it would be difficult to consider an acute schizophrenic state with elevated mood and blissful lack of intuition as a positive state of health". Nor is fitness enough: the fitness sought in athletic training is sometimes detrimental to physical health: what is needed is a 'minimalist' notion of fitness. Well-being, Downie suggests, requires both an essential reference to a good life and some conception of control over one's life. These factors, as well as the complex negative aspect, need to be considered when we ask ourselves what 'health' means.

Health is a graded, scalar, rather than dichotomous variable, and it can be and has been defined in countless ways. In fact, many of the measures used as indices of health status are not measures of health at all but of health service use (visits to health care providers (hospital admissions)).

In their seminal paper, R.N. Jadad and L. O'Grady point out that health can coexist with illness: it is possible to be sick and healthy at the same time. A Canadian survey of more than 3000 people aged 65 or older clearly illustrates this point, showing that 86% of people with one, 77% with two, and 51% with three or more diseases rated their health as good, very good or excellent. These data are replicated countless times in quality-of-life studies that include self-rated health. A meta-analysis of 22 cohort studies found that people who rated their health as poor had twice the risk of mortality as those who rated their health as excellent [309].

WHO surveys that assess an individual's health status ask questions about mobility, self-care, pain, cognition, interpersonal activities, vision, sleep, energy, and affect? The answers fall into a single metric ranging from dead (0) to perfect health (1)?

There are many indicators of health: oral health, reproductive and sexual health, mental health, injuries, and violence such as deaths from injuries or homicides, environmental quality, substance abuse, clinical prevention services, etc.

In fact, doctors are interested in diseases, not health, so that medical textbooks are a massive catalogue of diseases. The preferred view of health is the ability to adapt, self-manage and participate in social activities, including work. Sigmund Freud defined 'health' as the ability to love and work.

But if health is not an objective thing, a natural phenomenon, what is the meaning of the term 'health' and how can we make sense of it?

7.2 Health and the Philosophy of Medicine

Boorse supported a first descriptive and naturalistic approach [310]. An organism is healthy at any given time in proportion to its absence of disease, and disease is an internal state of the organism that interferes with the performance of a natural function, namely a typical contribution of the species to survival and reproduction. Naturalism does not correctly reflect our use of the term 'health' because it neglects the role that values play in determining whether someone is healthy or not. The notion of function is central to Boorse's approach and has attracted the most serious criticism even from those who are otherwise generally quite sympathetic to his descriptivism [311, 312]. Forced to explain the meaning of 'normal functioning', Boorse argued that normality is primarily a statistical construct guided by scientific hypotheses that rely on hard evidence about the functional levels typical of species. Yet species are not natural types or genera in biological taxonomy [313].

Natural genus theorists assume that the terms of natural genera reflect the divisions of nature, even though biological theory does not distinguish between natural and non-natural states.

More recently Jonathan Sholl edited a book in which sixty authors attempt unsuccessfully to define and/or explain the concept of health on biological grounds [314]. None of them define what they mean by health, so the sixty essays that make up the book share the term "health" and not the concept of health. There is no indication that they refer to the same concept.

The authors also fall victim to the common mistake of basing health on the concept of homeostasis. However, homeostasis is the essence of life and is found in the philosophical analysis of most issues relating to biology or disease (cancers are homeostatic systems). It would be rather surprising if it did not also contribute to the idea of health! But since there is nothing specific about this relationship, it is not definitional.

The editor, Jonathan Sholl, tends to believe that health is a natural state, but he adds that this concept does not lend itself to observation, which seems to indicate that it is not a scientific concept, but a philosophical one, i.e., hypothetical. If this is so, then the various uses of the term 'health' represent definitions that are not descriptive in nature but are speculative stipulations.

Philosophers of medicine distinguish between the properties of a thing that are essential to it and those that are merely accidental. They look for the primary element of the notion of health, its nature, or that without which it could not be what it is. However, 'health' admits of no authoritative definition, as it is essentially the subject of different narratives.

This book and its project represent a philosophical error which consists in trying to unify on biological grounds a heterogeneous set of biomedical situations which have nothing in common with each other, except for a vague psychosocial or existential concept. It is philosophical nonsense to try to find a biological answer to a family of disparate medical phenomena but brought together under the guise of a societal judgment. It is what Gilbert Ryle has called a category fallacy, in which things belonging to one category are presented as if they belonged to another, so that a property is attributed to something that could not possibly have that property.

Other authors rely more on the power of evolution or homeostasis to account for normal functioning.

Other authors rely more on the power of evolution or homeostasis to account for normal functioning [315, 316].

Nordenfelt has led a second normativist approach, arguing that health can only be understood philosophically if and until it is clear why it is valuable [317, 318]. Health is not simply a biological norm, it is an ideal. Health is about the ability to act and live life to the fullest and to achieve all one's vital goals.

Nordenfelt also rejected Boorse's biostatistical theory not because health is not rooted in biology, but because the mechanism that limits individual health cannot be identified in the same way as diseases or injuries are, simply because they result in statistically abnormal levels of biological functioning. What is important about health is that it is focused on what matters to the population in terms of their body and mental functioning, and this must in some sense connect analytically with human well-being. The philosophical debate between Boorse and Nordenfelt was at its peak from the late 1970s to the early 1990s [319].

Because of the enduring importance of the 1948 WHO definition, there has been a renewed interest in the normative conceptualization of health in recent years. Although some philosophers found common ground between the two approaches [320], others, particularly in the field of mental health, have argued that Boorse's natural functions approach cannot explain why mental illnesses are considered problematic [321].

For a normativist like Huber, the importance of coping and self-management plays a very different role in helping to explain the underlying human value that effective health interventions reinforce [322]. Huber and his colleagues include in their considerations the ability to participate in social activities including work.

The great English philosopher R.M. Hare has highlighted the difficulties of Boorse's views and supported an evaluative treatment of the concept of health [323].

However, limiting health to a standard is unsatisfactory, as this does not answer the obvious question of why anyone would care about normal functioning unless it is unpleasant, uncomfortable, painful, or generally negative to fall below the threshold.

Naturalism is the approach most likely to be accepted in the philosophy of medicine, but here again a divorce appears between the two disciplines, since medicine fails to satisfy the desideratum of being naturalistic. Normativism fails to achieve its desideratum of accurately describing how we use the terms 'health' and 'disease'. And the hybrid approach, which tries to combine the naturalistic and the normative approach, closes the discussion of controversial cases, and its naturalistic approach is not naturalistic.

This definition of health suffers from an important logical confusion, namely that it confuses cause and effect, i.e., the social determinants of health (e.g., unemployment rates, or other factors that limit an individual's effectiveness in achieving 'social health') with one of the components of the concept of health.

7.3 The Nature of Health

Who could claim to be in a state of complete physical, mental, and social well-being? Hardly anyone.

Health is therefore not a dichotomous system that allows only two alternatives but a scalar system. Good and bad health are part of a continuum. The assessment of health by the Karnofsky index, which goes in ten steps from 100 (perfect health) to zero (death), quantifies the level of health [324].

Many, if not most, people are in a continuous state of moderate sub-clinical illness. They are in these states of illness to the extent that they are not in an optimal state of health. We generally only apply the label 'disease' when we are so far from optimal health that specific symptoms manifest themselves. The manifestation of symptoms of disease is simply the lowest point on the scale at which one is most ill, i.e., furthest from health. In the biomedical sciences, however, one can understand a disease without prior knowledge of the idea of health.

However, health is the subject of a wild explosion of hypotheses which seek to define it, and which have little coherence between them if they are not contradictory. There is an amalgam of naturalistic or evaluative concepts; for some, health contributes to well-being, but for others, it does not. *The literature often confuses health with speculative causes such as natural selection, with physiological considerations or with social consequences in its search for a definition.*

Wittgenstein believed that, since traditional concepts of health care embody a concern for comfort and suffering, their entire purpose will not be fulfilled by the concepts of scientific medicine. The scientific goals of prediction and control are not the only respectable goals. As there is little consensus on the notion of health, this suggests, or confirms, that it is not a natural state amenable to a scientific approach, but a social, medical, and philosophical construct.

The word "health" is not a purely referential designator but a domain bringing together various applications that are overlapping. In its linguistic use, it is a continuum with no gaps in it, used in the social context of ordering, measuring, counting and so on. No clear dividing line exists between being healthy, being healthier and being labeled as unhealthy. There are gradients in health, which is a scalar concept [325].

Yet, beyond this descriptive account, it also conveys the speaker's approval of it. In fact, if anything belongs to the notion of 'health', it is that it is desirable, that it should happen, and this is not the result of anything factual. Even if health is not defined by well-being, it may be that what matters about the concept of health for practical purposes is its expression as well-being. There are practical, albeit imperfect, ways of measuring well-being through the measurement of preferences or through the measurement of subjective experience.

We should not seek to give a universal definition of health but determine different systems of rules corresponding to different language games that will be appropriately defined by usage. These language games are objects of comparison which by similarities and differences should shed light on the disparate facts of the use of the vague term health. They are not about ideas or about any essence of health, but rather about the functioning of speech acts. "*Rather than making the ideal 'an object of comparison—as it were, a standard', it is made 'a prejudice to which one must conform. This is the dogmatism into which philosophy so easily falls*" [326].

The different levels of aggregation of well-being characteristics then apply to a condition that is heterogeneous in nature because these different levels correspond to different concepts of health. Health is a concept of family resemblances. Wittgenstein showed that objects designated by a term can be related to each other, not by a common property or essence, but by a network of similarities, like people whose faces share characteristic family features.

A range of positive and negative social, psychological, and environmental factors have a powerful influence on physical and mental health. The central problem is that health has a negative and a positive dimension.

On the one hand, the exposures that increase the risk of disease are important: poor diet, lack of exercise, pollution, smoking, insufficient sleep, menopause, epidemics, etc.

On the other hand, neglecting the positive assets of health gives an impoverished picture of the determinants of health at the population level. What people consider essential to well-being is a matter of character, defined as moral excellence and long considered central to well-being. The term "flourishing", used for thousands of years and literally meaning "to grow" or "to prosper", represents a powerful way of looking at health in its broadest sense.

William Jenner pointed out, that there is no health as such, since the determination of what health means depends on our goals, our horizons, our energies, our impulses and our mistakes; there are innumerable health's of the body, and "the more we set aside the dogma of 'the equality of men', the more the concept of normal health, as well as the concept of normal diet and the normal course of a disease, must be abandoned by our physicians. Only then would it be time to consider the health and sickness of the soul: in the case of one person, health might, of course, resemble the opposite of health in another person".

Bognat and Hirose write: "*In the end, we do not care much about health itself. What we care about is its value to us. What we care about is how it affects our well-being and the quality of our lives*" [327]. Broome states that, "*The value of a health condition to an individual is the extent to which it promotes or diminishes their well-being*" [328].

The Director-General of the World Health Organization, Tedros Ghebreyesus Organization, Tedros Ghebreyesus, has announced that leaders of major economies will discuss a "*One Health*" strategy at the upcoming G7 and G20 meetings.

We cannot protect human health without addressing the impact of human activities that disrupt ecosystems, encroach on habitats, and promote climate change. One option could be to use a One Health calculator as an addition to GDP.

One Health is a term used to describe the inextricable links between human, animal, plant and environmental health and ecosystems. A One Health calculator could measure the state of a nation's natural resources, the purity of its environment, the biodiversity of its ecosystem, the sustainability of its agriculture, the health of its flora and fauna, the resilience of its food security, and the life expectancy of its population.

Tyler Vanderweele of the Harvard School of Public Health has proposed a brief framework for what he calls "positive epidemiology" including: (1) happiness and life satisfaction; (2) self-rated physical and mental health; (3) meaning and purpose; (4) character and virtue; (5) close social relationships; (6) financial security [329].

We need a positive epidemiology to understand the full range of health assets, not just the traditional risk factors. We need positive epidemiology because, both in terms of data and methodology, this discipline has enormous potential to contribute even more to the flourishing of all humanity.

7.4 What Do We Mean by 'Health'?

The concept of health has multiple meanings depending on how it is used. None of them is true, because it is a series of conventions which, each of them has its use: absence of disease; complex fact of physical, mental and social well-being; a state that medicine seeks to restore; a measurable scalar variable that represents a continuum between maximum health and zero health; an intrinsically positively valid state; a natural, biological, physiological and tangible state; a holistic state laden with values (the main purposes, meaning and purposes of life); according to Freud, the capacity to love and to work; there are several specific health concepts, such as food health, sexual health, oral health, etc. Defining health recalls Saint Agustín of Hippo who said about time: "*What is time? If no one asks me, I know. If I want to explain it to anyone who asks me, I don't know anymore*".

Wittgenstein asserted that the meaning of words depends on their use. What he meant was that depending on what one might call their function (which includes an infinite variety of uses, for example, designating an object or saying what one thinks) and depending on their context of use (which can be scientific, poetic, colloquial, etc.), words can function in totally different ways. The meaning of a word cannot be determined in the same way for each use case of a word. For example, the word "apple" normally refers to a fruit, but it is context sensitive: "the big apple" is the name of New York City.

In contrast, the word "health" does not usually refer to a physical or natural object as the word "apple" does. We can change the meaning of this word, but then it would no longer correspond to the same concept [330].

Let us conclude with Quentin Crisp that health is about having the same disease as your neighbors.

Chapter 8
Causality

Felix qui potuit rerum cognoscere causas

Virgil

Abstract Diseases depend on a causal network. Causes are dispositions characterized by the strength of association, their plausibility, their manipulability, the probability increase, and their counterfactual dependence, although absence may be included in causal claims. Epidemiology measures trends towards sufficiency and necessity. Causal pluralism may be analysed in terms of structural equations. There are causal and manifestational diseases. Randomized controlled trials provide a rigorous tool to examine cause-effect relationships.

Risk factors are factors associated with an increased probability of an unfavourable outcome, that is potentially but not necessarily a causal factor.

Keywords Causality · Capacities · INUS · Necessary and/or sufficient · Manipulability · Probability increase · Counterfactual dependence · Reverse causality · Structural model · Causal and manifestational diseases · Randomized control trials · Risks · Genetics

The main objective of epidemiology is to identify the alterable causes of disease [331].

Long-standing philosophical problems concern the nature of the cause and how we discover it. Hume argued that a supposed 'power' of *A* to bring about *B* 'necessarily' is not empirical, so that this idea is illegitimate; all we can observe is that *A*'s have been consistently followed by *B*s in the past. Critics object that this does not distinguish between causal connections and mere accidental but universal regularities [332].

Imagine the death of a person who describes herself as caused by lung cancer. Lung cancer may be caused by a genetic mutation or by repeated deposition of carcinogens in the lung tissue, itself caused by smoking. Smoking, in turn, was probably caused by the smoker's propensity for addictive behaviour, peer pressure and the socio-economic environment. Which of the many candidate hypotheses of

L. Karhausen, *The Fragility of Philosophy of Medicine*, Philosophy and Medicine 147, https://doi.org/10.1007/978-3-031-41633-0_8

the form "*A* caused *B*" (where *B* represents the death of the patient) best explains the outcome? There is hardly an absolute answer to this question.

What makes a certain causality in medicine adequate is either our ability or the need to intervene on the factor in question. The accumulation of carcinogens in lung tissue can be prevented by not smoking. On the other hand, while it is not yet possible to prevent the mutations associated with the different subtypes of cancer, medical research is striving to develop targeted therapies and interventions to control and prevent their consequences [333].

The role of analytical epidemiology is to identify the modifiable causes of disease and to describe the Baconian notion of its natural history. Epidemiology is not simply "the study of the frequency of disease and the distribution of health states in human populations" [334], but "*the study of the distribution and determinants of disease frequency in human populations*" [335]. Epidemiology is therefore not purely descriptive but plays a major role in establishing causal relationships [336].

Nancy Cartwright in her original work on causality [337] has argued that causal claims are *capacities,* i.e., potentialities, which she sometimes calls tendencies. Causality is not a single thing, as is commonly believed. There is a wide variety of causal relationships, each with different characteristics, different methods of discovery and different uses. Causal chains represent only a fraction of reality, and the whole should more appropriately be seen as a network, the complexity of which is far beyond our understanding.

That causality is a necessary connection is an idea that goes back to Aristotle's Metaphysics, an idea very common among philosophers of the past. Causality, in this view, is seen as a relationship of a logical nature.

"*When agent and patient meet according to their powers, one acts, and the other is influenced by Necessity... That which has rational power (e.g., medical knowledge, which can kill or cure) necessarily does what it has the power to do and as it has the power, when it has the desire to do so*" [338].

It is this Aristotelian way of seeing that David Hume reverses: he rejects the logical nature of the causal relation, without rejecting its apparent necessity. David Hume insists that it is not possible in a single case, when *A* is the cause of *B*, to find the necessary connecting element between *A* and *B*. What we observe, he says, is simply *A* followed by *B*, but we do not observe 'any quality that links the effect to the cause'.

Where then do we get the idea of the 'necessary connection' of the causal 'must'? We get it, says Hume, from the observation of many similar cases where *A*s are followed by *Bs*. These repeated observations have the effect of creating a 'connection ... which we feel in the mind'.

Wittgenstein notes that this conclusion may seem surprising: "*My views will be regarded by many as extravagant or ridiculous. What? The effectiveness of a cause lies in the determination of the mind! As if causes did not operate completely independently of the mind...*" [339].

Kant, in turn, impressed by Hume's discovery, seeks to establish an a priori conception of causality that proceeds according to a rule. If the connection between events of type A and events of type B is strictly universal and consists in conformity with a rule, then we could have no empirical grounds for affirming it. We can only make such judgements if we believe that there is a necessary connection between *A* and *B* that allows us to venture beyond the limit of our observations.

How is this possible? How can a statement be true, i.e., true of the world, and yet not be subject to refutation by eventual or possible experience of the world? We generally think that our knowledge must be 'true to reality'. Indeed, it must, says Kant, but it is also true that 'objects must conform to our knowledge'.

Do our mental faculties determine the way the world is? Or does the world conform to our wishes and demands? No, Kant replies, the world as we perceive it through our senses, and as we understand it through our reason, must be adapted to our mode of perception and cognition. It is not the world 'as it is in itself' that we perceive, but the world filtered through our senses and our understanding.

In other words, causality for Kant is not, as for Hume, a mere associative attitude, but a fundamental form of our understanding, and is therefore not a component of reality. There is no causal ontology in Kant. Kant's transcendentalism attributes the omnipresence of causal extrapolations from immutable categories, a priori to the intellect.

Wittgenstein does not deny that events have causes, but he is careful not to go too far in believing in causality [340]. "There are causes, but there is no reason to believe that all events are part of an interconnected network. There is no cause as a necessary connection between two events, no cause that requires its effect. The only necessity is logical, not causal.

One could say, writes Elizabeth Anscombe, that everything is determined once it has happened. This inversion of the order of things explains the causal theory of INUS: John Mackie introduced this term in 1960 (insufficient, but necessary part of an unnecessary but sufficient condition).

Rothmann, who is a determinist, introduced into epidemiology the idea of INUS, which he borrowed from J.L. Mackie [341], i.e., that a cause is an insufficient but necessary part of a condition, which is itself unnecessary but sufficient for the outcome [342]. The concept may eventually be useful for thinking about the relationship between component causes, i.e. whether the joint effect of two component causes would be different if they were members of the same causal constellation or not. However, we have so little information about the different causes of the same disease that it is difficult to assess the usefulness of this speculative and deterministic model. As for the term "necessary cause" in this context, we do not even know if there is a single disease for which we know when this goal was achieved, except when necessity, the term "necessary" is used in the INUS sense, i.e., retrospectively, when the die is cast [343].

In the *Philosophical Investigations*, the reader is invited to consider our practice of calling something a reason and to describe the conditions for the correct application of the concept. Whereas Kant sees causality as a universal category of our descriptions, Wittgenstein sees it as a fact about our descriptions, traceable to the practice of language games and closer to scapegoating than to science [344]. Causality is not a cognitive lamp with which rational beings illuminate the world. It is a tacit presupposition that circumscribes human linguistic activity in circumstances that are primarily social. These presuppositions are neither transcendental nor conceptual but are essentially practical or adaptive.

Wittgenstein explains the role of causality in science by a neo-Kantian version of causal laws. What he points to is a certain 'form of description' that is crucial for scientific theorization. Wittgenstein does not abandon the Kantian idea that descriptions of the world are conceivable only in terms of causality but rejects the claim that this is so because there are unchanging logical categories underlying the relation of language to the world. Causality is a principle that takes the form of real logical laws, but it is not a law, but the form of a law [345].

The principle of causality according to which every event must have a cause is therefore not an a priori synthetic statement as Kant thought, but a disguised rule of grammar, that is, a rule of language [346]. The source of necessity would lie solely in language. If this means that our grammar simply excludes the expression 'uncaused event' as absurd, this is wrong. It is rather a standard of representation of classical mechanics.

Causal propositions, for Wittgenstein, are unquestionable not because they are solidly based on a priori categories or intuitions, but because there is no question of them not being based. We cannot be certain of any specific cause, but we must be certain that there is a cause in general. When something happens, we look for the cause. The grammar of causality is not based on scientific facts, logical categories, or indirect intuitions. The idea that there is an irreducible variety of types of causality, and that the notion of non-necessary causes is rooted in the lever of action rather than observation, is central to determining the choice of medical interventions. To know is to give a verdict [347].

The search for causes is a non-scientific, eminently practical matter. "*... to call something a cause is to point to someone and say, 'he did it'*" [348]. The search for a cause is a human reaction to the social facts of life. We do not observe causal relations, we do not project causality into the world, and we do not experience it intuitively: we proclaim it.

The simplest form of the causality game, for example in medicine, is the search for a scapegoat, guilty of all ills, even and especially when the trajectory of the emergence of the disease or illness in question is poorly known or unknown: it is a matter of finding a cause at all costs. We believe that there is a cause for every effect, so that causality in its scientific sense means predicting the effect from the cause. In contrast, the Darwinian interpretation, according to Wittgenstein, is to follow the cause from its effects [349].

Like Hume, Wittgenstein considers the causal relationship to be contingent and external, i.e., it is obtained between logically independent events [350, 351]. It is established empirically through observation and induction [352].

For Wittgenstein, causal relations are concepts of family resemblance that refuse analysis in terms of necessary and sufficient conditions. The claim that the only form of necessity is logical necessity must be replaced by a catalogue of different uses of the term necessity which in turn reveal different but interrelated meanings [353, 354].

8.1 Types of Causal Relationships

1. *necessary but not sufficient cause*

In this situation, a factor is necessary, but not sufficient, to cause the disease, as in the case of the tuberculosis bacillus

2. *sufficient but not necessary cause*

The factor alone can produce the disease, but also other factors acting alone (e.g., exposure to radiation and benzene can produce leukemia).

3. *neither sufficient nor necessary cause*

This is a more complex model, which more accurately represents the cause-and-effect relationship that operates in most chronic diseases.

The term cause has different meanings in different contexts.

Causality is presented as a system of similarities such as

1. The presence of the set of characteristics (the set of clusters) is sufficient to apply the concept.
2. No features are necessary.
3. At least one of the features must be instantiated.

In saying this, the multiple criteria for the use of the term causality does not mean that the term has multiple meanings. There are several overlapping characteristics of causality and none of them are common to all:

1. *Constant conjunction.*
   Our knowledge of causes, according to David Hume, does not result from demonstrative reasoning, but from what simply happens, namely the constant conjunction of two events, namely by the mere habit of expecting one when the other appears. Thus, if many instances of an isolated sequence 'A followed by B' have been repeatedly observed, they tend to be declared causally linked by a determining habit.
2. *Strength of association*
   The strength of the association is measured by the relative risk or odds ratio.
3. *Replication of results*
   If the relationship is causal, one would expect to find it consistently in different studies and in different populations.
4. *Plausibility and biological consistency*
   It is helpful if the relationship is biologically plausible and not inconsistent with known facts about the biology of the disease.
5. *Manipulability*
   The cause of a disease is the handle, so to speak, by which human beings can manipulate it [355].

An alteration in the frequency or quality of category A is followed by a change in another category B.

One of the aims of epidemiology is to identify the alterable causes of disease, namely those by the manipulation of which we can produce or prevent their abnormal or pathological effect. Manipulative causation assumes that we know what will happen if we do not intervene [356].

However, manipulability is not an essential condition of causality. Assumed causal relationships in the demographic domain of age, gender, race and ethnic group, or marital status are not manipulable. Nevertheless, the belief that the presumed effect would change if the cause changed is the concept that defines the causal relationship. The term *determinant* proposed in 1970 by Brian MacMahon is now used in epidemiology to cover both manipulable and non-manipulable factors. The latter, such as age, sex, occupation, and socio-economic level, are considered as proxies for manipulable causes. Determinants therefore have a broader scope than causal factors, as they are part of the medical explanation while they are closely linked to preventive or therapeutic interventions.

6. *Probability increase*

"Probabilistic causation" refers to a group of theories that aim to characterize the relationship between cause and effect using the tools of probability theory. The central idea of these theories is that causes change the probabilities of their effects, all else being equal [357].

Causality must be analyzed in probabilistic terms because causes make their effects more likely and revolve around the transmission of probabilities within ordered pairs of events: causality is a transmission of probability distributions [358].

Clinicians, epidemiologists, and medical scientists are methodologically probabilistic while often retaining a largely deterministic implicit approach [359].

We say that *A* causes *B* in each situation if and only if, in that situation, the probability of *B* conditional on *A* is greater than the probability of B conditional on non-*A*:

If *A*j represents a relevant contextual factor, we can define a cause *A* of a condition *B* as follows:

A is a positive cause of *B* if and only if:
P (*B*|*A* & *A*j) > P (*B*|non-*A* & *A*j) for all j.

7. *Counterfactual dependence*

In seeking to define causality as a constant conjunction, Hume added a second criterion: "or, in other words, if the first object had not been, the second never existed." Similarly, for Galileo, "once the cause takes place, the effect follows; and removed, the effect is removed" [360].

This second definition goes beyond the constant conjunction and corresponds to what logicians call contrary-to-fact conditionals, counterfactual conditionals, or subjunctive conditionals [361].

It is commonly accepted that there are two fundamentally different varieties of conditionals, the indicative, and the subjunctive. This distinction is marked by differences in grammatical mode. In indicative conditionals, the consequent verb is in the indicative, while in subjunctive conditionals it is in the subjunctive.

The following two sentences show the difference:

(1) If Oswald didn't shoot Kennedy, someone else did (indicative)
(2) If Oswald didn't shoot Kennedy, someone else would have. (Subjunctive)

To understand the difference, we need to ask what the evidence would be for each. If we think that Kennedy was indeed shot, then we would accept (1) without any further evidence. We know that someone shot him. If it wasn't Oswald, then it must have been someone else.

On the other hand, knowing that Kennedy was killed is not enough to accept (2). One could accept (2) if one had evidence that Oswald did not act alone but was part of a larger conspiracy, or if one thought that so many people wanted to kill Kennedy that someone else would have come forward. But if one thinks that the hypothesis that Oswald was alone is an anomaly, then one must reject (2).

Because it might be rational to accept (1) and reject (2), these two hypotheses would seem to have different truth conditions. (2) concerns what would have happened in a possible scenario where Oswald did not shoot Kennedy (if in fact Oswald did shoot Kennedy, then this scenario is a counterfactual, an alternative "possible world"). (1) however, concerns what happened in the world as it is.

Subjunctive conditionals are often called counterfactual conditionals because their antecedents are presented as contrary to the facts. But a counterfactual conditional is not a conditional with a false antecedent, and an indicative conditional with a true antecedent.

A counterfactual conditional may have a true antecedent (suppose Sylvia wrongly thinks she forgot to take her paracetamol to prevent her menstrual migraine and says: "If I had taken my painkiller, I wouldn't have had this migraine"). And an indicative conditional can have a false antecedent, as in (1). Yet it would be odd to assert a counterfactual that is known to have a true antecedent, or an indicative that is known to have a false antecedent, and any account of the difference between indicatives and subjunctives should explain this fact.

A counterfactual is a conditional statement, i.e., of the form if A, then B, whose antecedent is false. An important and controversial problem in logic concerns the truth conditions for counterfactuals.

A counterfactual model of causality also exists in philosophy, originating in David Lewis' seminal 1973 book *Counterfactuals* [362].

That said, subjunctive conditionals are not material conditionals. After all, we usually use them when we know that the antecedent is false. In these cases, the corresponding material conditional is always true. Indeed, material implication conditionals '$p \supset q$' are only false if p is true and q is false, so they are guaranteed to be true, whenever p is false, no matter what q says.

In contrast, since David Hume, deterministic causal statements, 'p causes q', are then equivalent to: (1) p is true (2) q is true and (3) if p were false, then q would be false, if all else remains unchanged.

In terms of counterfactual dependence, a causal chain is expressed as follows: p causes q, if and only if, if p had not occurred, then q would not have occurred.

However, in formal logic, counterfactuals seem to be true, vacuously true, since if p happens then q happens, but p does not. Therefore, counterfactuals are conditionals that are not verifiable, since their antecedent is subjunctive and therefore modal, so they fall under modal logic.

In sum, in predicative logic, the statement ‘p ⊃ q’ is verifiable and therefore obeys a truth table.

In contrast, counterfactual statements are represented in modal logic as follows:

‘ $\Box(\neg p \rightarrow q)$’, which means that if p had not happened, q would not have happened (where □ is called ‘a necessity’). The antecedent does not imply the consequent since it is contingently possible for the antecedent to be true and the consequent false. Counterfactual statements are therefore not verifiable.

8. *Preference for a proximal rather than a distant cause*

If we start to consider remote causes, we may never stop.

9. *Causation by absence*

Absence can be included in causal claims on both the cause-and-effect sides. Omissions and prevention are types of causation. A negative causal factor (e.g., a preventive factor) is either a positive causal factor for not-B, or it will be represented by the same expression where the sign < is substituted for the sign >:

$P(B|A \& K) < (B|K)$.

For an irrelevant causal factor, the = sign will be substituted for the > sign: $P(B|A \& K) = (B|K)$.

Lack of vitamin B12 is the cause of pernicious anemia, and this disease is successfully treated with vitamin B12 injections.

10. *The causal network*

MacMahon called the *Web of Causation* [363]. Effects do not depend on single causes and the concept of a causal chain, while useful, has the defect of being too simplistic. Causality is usually the result of a web of broad classes of events, so that each component is the result of a myriad of effects of those components. The whole causal framework should be seen as a network whose complexity is far beyond our understanding, and many such networks may exist for a given disease [364]. More recently, this idea has been taken up in philosophy of medicine under the label of the causal mosaic [365].

11. *Reverse causality*

Reverse causation means that X and Y are associated, but not in the way one might expect. Instead of X causing a change in Y, the opposite happens: Y causes changes in X. In epidemiology, the exposure-disease process is then reversed; in other words, the disease causes the risk factor. Thus, because Y unexpectedly precedes X, the reverse causality bias is sometimes called the "cart before the horse" bias.

For example, low social status is a cause of schizophrenia, but schizophrenia is a cause of downward social mobility.

Or, about physical activity and CHD, it is essential to check that some early CHD symptoms (before a diagnosis is possible) have not altered the patient's exercise habits; for example, having difficulty breathing when climbing stairs could reduce or prevent exercise, so the disease could have caused the change in the risk factor—a reverse causation phenomenon.

12. *Beware of selective publications*

Outcome-based selection occurs when reviewers and editors allow recommendations and publication decisions to depend on study results rather than on the transparency and robustness of methods and data collection. Publication bias distorts the medical literature [366].

8.2 The Unnatural Nature of Causation

Causal processes linking cause and effect are a thorny issue. Hilary Putnam writes: "The materialist metaphysician often takes the causal relationship as an example of an embedded structure." It is true that philosophers who think from the armchair find themselves embarrassed by the complexity of life forms represented by medical interventions. This is probably why they prefer to avoid the subject.

On the one hand, if one assumes that the description of the world in science in general, as well as in medicine, is mind-independent, it could be given in purely physicalist terms. Yet, in this case, intentionality cannot be in the physical domain. In so-called epistemic naturalism, events have causes and objects have causal powers, and the causes are in the world itself, they are constructed in the world itself. Causal relation.

But for another, Hilary Putnam argues that 'the cause' is roughly 'that part of the total cause which can reasonably, given contextually appropriate interests, be regarded as the trigger as opposed to a background condition, and thus that the concept of "the cause" implies something intentional' [367].

Putnam adds that the fact that something, such as a causal relationship, is interesting in relation to something intentional does not mean that it is non-objective. It follows that the search for causes in medicine or epidemiology "smuggles in intentional/semantic notions". In this respect, causality, like truth, is an intentional and contextual notion that depends on the specific interest and salient points of the researchers, not a 'view from nowhere'.

Kant saw causality as a feature of experience, but he was reluctant to admit the existence of causes in the world outside our experience of it. Causes are not to be understood as actually existing properties, such as mass, weight, or other natural properties.

Mackie argued that causality is epistemic, not something in the world. They are like tickets of inference, to quote Gilbert Ryle, that allow us to move from one assertion to another, which is not the same as arguing that there is a special, occult force or hidden property that is responsible for this change. Danto concludes that the question of whether the world is causally ordered apart from the way we think about it is almost a meaningless question. Perhaps the principle of causality is not a statement about the world, nor something we learn from the world, but something we bring to the world.

In this context, it is not difficult to appreciate how Nancy Cartwright gets us out of this dilemma with her seminal book *Hunting Causes and Using Them* [368]. According to her, causality is a label we use to classify various events and processes such as 'causes', 'enables', 'helps', 'allows', 'forces', 'requires', 'allows', 'helps', 'inhibits', 'prevents', etc. Cause is a plural concept. Different accounts of causality seem to disagree with each other only because the same word has different meanings in different contexts.

"*Causal laws cannot be suppressed, as they are necessary to ground the distinction between effective and ineffective strategies*," writes Cartwright.

For an epidemiologist or physician, causal claims are nothing beyond their evidence or the collection of that evidence. The meaning of a causal assertion is identified with its verification, writes Arthur Danto [369]: "the concept of causality dissolves in the evidence we have for it". That is, epidemiological methods provide an implicit definition of causality in epidemiology. However, the best definition of causality in medicine lies in the methods of analytical epidemiology.

The progressive methodological sophistication of the last 40 years is perfectly in line with a progressive implicit recasting of our concept of causality. Any definition of causality in medicine therefore inevitably dissolves in the use of epidemiological methods and the process of methodological revisions leads to implicit or explicit, partial, or complete re-examinations of our concept of causality. Thus, specifying the use of the term cause does not tell us what it means.

"All events in the material world and in biology are produced by chains of causes. However, if causality were an intrinsic property of nature, a material necessity that connects all events in the material world, it might be justified to regard our actions as mere links in a causal network that weaves itself continuously from the Big Bang to the Big Crunch" [370].

8.3 Epidemiology: Trends Towards Sufficiency and Necessity

Analytical epidemiology, as opposed to descriptive epidemiology, seeks to identify the determinants of disease processes. While the cohort study looks at the frequency of disease in exposed and unexposed individuals, the case-control study looks at the frequency and degree of exposure in individuals with a specific disease (cases) and those without the disease (controls).

The *cohort study* design identifies a group of people exposed to a particular factor and a control group that has not been exposed to that factor, and then measures and compares the incidence of disease in the two groups. A higher incidence of disease in the exposed group suggests an association between that factor and the disease outcome. This type of study is generally a good choice when dealing with a disease in a relatively small and well-defined source population, especially if the disease being studied is common.

The *case-control study* design uses a different sampling strategy in which researchers identify a group of individuals who have developed the disease (the cases) and a control group of individuals who have not had the disease in question (the controls). Cases and controls are then compared according to the frequency of one or more past exposures. If cases have a significantly higher probability of exposure to a particular factor than controls, this suggests an association. This strategy is a better choice when the source population is large and ill-defined and is particularly useful when the disease outcome is uncommon.

The issue is that, since we reject necessary and sufficient causes, necessity and sufficiency become limiting concepts that express tendencies towards necessity or sufficiency. In fact, case-control studies measure the tendency towards necessity, and cohort studies the tendency towards sufficiency.

Causal tendencies, according to John Stuart Mill, do not indicate what effect occurs when the cause is present, but rather what the cause contributes to an effect in more realistic circumstances where other relevant causal factors have not been eliminated. Cartwright defends the view that causal assertions are really assertions of capacity or tendency, i.e. local checkers [371].

There are degrees of causal sufficiency and degrees of causal necessity [372].

If C (cause) tends to produce E (effect), then:

(1) The probability of sufficiency is, as it were, prospective: it is the probability that C produces E in a situation where there are no other causes of E present, and C and E are absent.
(2) The probability of necessity is retrospective: it is the probability that E would not have occurred in the absence of C, given that C and E did occur.

We now turn to David Hume's two questions about causality.

First, is C regularly followed by E?

Cohort studies ask this question with a modifier: to what extent is C regularly followed by E? Then, C is a positive cause for E means that E is more likely given C, than in the absence of C. C is considered to have a positive statistical relationship with E. If this is the case, in the hypothetical exposed population, where all individuals would be exposed to C, there would be a certain percentage of individuals with the E effect that reflects the probability P (E|C).

The higher this probability, the more C becomes a sufficient condition. This probability of C being sufficient is a random variable with a numerical value in the closed interval [1, 0]: namely with a value of 1 when E is present and 0 when it is absent. Therefore, in the unexposed counterfactual population, there will be a certain percentage of individuals with the E effect.

Thus, the results generally lie on a continuum between the two extremes, sufficiency, and necessity.

In the case of sufficiency, at one end, P (E|C) = 1 in the hypothetical exposed group. And at the other end of the spectrum, we would have: P (E|non-C) = 0 in the counterfactual control group. This means that the causal contribution of C increases if C tends towards sufficiency. The lower the percentage of unexposed subjects in the contrast group, the closer C is to sufficiency. If there are no unexposed subjects, C is necessary.

In the light of the above, C has a tendency towards sufficiency if and only if the conditional probability of E given C is greater than the conditional probability of E given non-C; at the end of the spectrum, in the case of sufficiency, E and C are absent. The tendency of C to the sufficiency of E (attributable risk) can therefore be measured by the difference between two conditional probabilities: P (E|C) − P (E| non-C). Its value varies from 0 to 1, i.e., from causal irrelevance to causal quasi-determinism. The higher the difference, the more sufficient C is found to be.

Second, case-control studies raise Hume's second question, "if the first object had not been, the second would never have existed [...]" with the same modifier: to what extent can the absence of E be predicted from the absence of C? Or, to what extent can the presence of C be predicted from the presence of E?

Case-control studies are concerned with the probability of finding a putative contributing cause given that the disease occurred. This probability P (C|E) also has a full range of degrees. The higher the percentage of exposed subjects in the hypothetical study group, the closer C is to necessity and vice versa: it thus measures the probability of necessity. In contrast, the lower the percentage of exposed subjects in the control group, the closer C is to sufficiency. If C is absent in the control population, C is sufficient for E.

Thus, C has a tendency towards sufficiency for E if and only if the conditional probability of C given E is greater than that of C in the absence of E, in the case where the disease and exposure occurred. The following difference measures the tendency for C to be necessary for E:

P (C|E) − P (C Non-E)

If it is not statistically significant, C is not causally relevant to E.

The above allows the view, details, and objections aside, that cohort studies are of the form: if C is a contributing cause of E, C, as an alternative to non-C, would tend to be a sufficient condition for E. And case-control studies specify the alternative: if E rather than non-E had occurred, C (the putative cause) would tend to be a necessary condition.

In short, cohort studies measure causal trends towards sufficiency, and case-control studies measure trends towards necessity. In any case, if we abandon determinism, sufficiency and necessity become limiting concepts.

8.4 Judea Pearl and Structural Equations

In her seminal book, Judea Pearl rejects causal pluralism and defends a substantive theory of causality, defined, analyzed, and formulated in her structural causal models (SCMs) [373]. Presenting the probability calculus as a set of logical propositions, he brings together with unique impact a probabilistic and counterfactual approach to causality and the effects of potential interventions. As such, it conceives of causality in terms of a causal diagram.

To evaluate the sentences of this logical system, it uses causal structures modelled by Bayes networks, with sets of arrows expressing a certain hypothesis about what affects what. The resulting toolkit visually summarizes the theory with diagrams, using "directed acyclic graphs" (DAGs) which, when drawn, connect (cause) nodes (variables) together. DAGs consist of single-headed arrows, so that no variable can cause itself. The absence of arrows between two variables indicates that it is assumed that there is no causal relationship between them. Pearl's logic language allows conditionals in the indicative and subjunctive tenses. If this is the case, then the causality graphs show when one factor would increase the responsibility of another variable. It shows not only what happens, but also what would happen if something else happened.

It is only recently that epidemiology and science in general have acquired the mathematical language of statistics. Harvard professor Gary King puts this revolution into historical perspective: "More has been learned about causal inference in the last few decades than the sum of all that had been learned about it in all of previous history. Judea Pearl's book explains how to define causal parameters; it highlights the assumptions needed to estimate causal parameters in a variety of situations, whether they have testable implications, and how to predict the effects of interventions and reason counterfactually [374].

8.5 Nancy Cartwright and Family Resemblances

The concept of causality refers to a whole family of relationships or syntactic structures. Causal relations are not sui generis, are not reducible to non-causal relations, and have no distinctive features. The specific causal verbs to which Nancy Cartwright draws attention—attract, repel, raise, feel, lower, break, and so on—are non-specific and uninformative [375].

The statement that all diseases have a cause is grammatical in nature.

In some cases, causality has a special character. Some causes are extrinsic to the organism, such as infections or trauma, others are intrinsic, such as genetic diseases, such as those due to congenital malformation, or placebos and nocebos. Co-morbidity can be another form of causation, for example when nephrosclerosis and its associated high blood pressure cause cardiovascular disease or when gingivitis increases the risk of Alzheimer's disease.

Some causes are dispositions. A disposition, in philosophy, is a property whose presence or absence would only manifest itself—make an observable difference—under certain conditions. Fragility is a dispositional property: to say that an object is fragile is to say that it will break if struck with sufficient force. Two pieces of metal, only one of which is brittle, may look identical. The difference will only be revealed if both are struck.

The risk of schizophrenia is increased in certain circumstances, including various obstetric complications, urban birth or residence, famines, migrant status, and seasonal effects via prenatal infections, such as influenza [376]. In other words, the various genetic factors of schizophrenia are sometimes dispositions that are revealed by environmental factors.

Nancy Cartwright questions whether there is a method of causal inference that is applicable to all cases and, in contrast to Pearl in epidemiology, advocates causal pluralism. Under the influence of Hume and Kant, causality is often seen as a monolithic concept. She believes that there are in fact a variety of causal relationships that operate in different ways and that a variety of different questions can be asked. She also questions one of Pearl's assumptions, that it is possible to change causal relationships in one part of the system while leaving causal links unchanged elsewhere. She adds that Bayes network methods do not apply, for example, when the positive and negative effects of a single factor cancel each other out, when factors can follow the same time trend without being causally linked, or when populations with different causal structures or probability measures are mixed.

8.6 Causal Diseases

The term "disease" is vague, as it depends on the criteria one decides to use to separate pathology from physiology, and in any case, there is no clear dividing line between its applicability and non-applicability. There is a multiplicity of definitional criteria as well as a multiplicity of meanings for the use of the word, and there is no single, defined set of conditions governing its use. It is not surprising, therefore, that the question of who is ill and who is not rarely arises in hospital wards but is not properly applicable to populations where illnesses exist as a qualitative continuum.

However, Brian MacMahon [377] has identified two ways of classifying sick people: diseases can be interpreted in purely descriptive terms, or in terms of their etiology, i.e., causative diseases. Two types of criteria are used to categorize sick people.

1. *Manifestation criteria*: sick people are grouped according to similarity of symptoms, signs, changes in body or tissue chemistry, behaviour, prognosis, or a combination of these characteristics. Examples are fractures, diabetes mellitus, mental retardation, the common cold, schizophrenia, and breast cancer.

2. *Causal criteria*: Causal grouping depends on the similarity of individuals with respect to one or more experiences that are thought to cause their disease. Examples of diseases defined by causal criteria are birth trauma, silicosis, syphilis, lead poisoning, Covid-19.

Morton Beckner called them polytypic and monotypic, but *polythetic* and *monothetic* might be more appropriate terms [378].

Single-criteria diseases are an entirely different group of diseases from those defined by manifestations and *family resemblances*; they have a necessary and sufficient criterion for identification that are referential in nature, as are proper names.

Causal diseases are a sub-category of single-criteria diseases, known since Galen. Their definition is given by denotation, i.e., in terms of a single, proximal, specific, a posteriori, and consequently necessary and sufficient cause (or causal process). A thing is a scar if an injury caused it.

Disease designators in the case of causal diseases would be called *rigid designators* by the philosopher and logician Saul Kripke [379], professor at New York University, because they are purely and necessarily referential; they are attached to the world by stipulation, because the causal link between the world and language is not empirical but lexical. There are certain types of words that resist family resemblance or have very small families. This phenomenon is called rigidity. Technical or scientific sounding words often cause this phenomenon. Disease designators in the case of causal diseases are therefore not necessary but a priori.

The shift from a descriptive to an etiological and referential taxonomy in the case where it is either microbiological (infectious diseases), nutritional (scurvy) or genetic reveals the philosopher's stone of medicine, namely the hope of absorbing all diseases into causal diseases; it is a quest for cognitive coherence and intelligibility.

As a result, causal disorders represent stipulative decisions created by medicine and adopted by medical grammar. A clear boundary is imposed. The causes of monocriteria disorders are not contingent facts, like scientific causes, but are a priori necessarily true and contain the counterfactual assumption that when the cause is not present, there is no disease.

However, the crucial step and the most original and interesting idea of Kripke here is to radically dissociate the two traditionally confused notions of necessity and apriority. The *necessary/contingent* distinction belongs to metaphysics, and the *a priori/a posteriori* distinction to epistemology. From the fact that a statement is necessary (true in all possible worlds), it does not automatically follow that its truth can be known a priori (independently of any experience). Kripke is, in any case, right to point out that this conclusion is not self-evident and would need to be really justified. There is not necessarily a contradiction between the fact that 'a b' is a necessary identity and the fact that the recognition of this identity must be the subject of empirical discovery.

Disease designators in the case of causal diseases are therefore not necessary but a priori.

The shift from a descriptive to an etiological and referential taxonomy in the case where it is either microbiological (infectious diseases), nutritional (scurvy) or genetic reveals the philosopher's stone of medicine, namely the hope of absorbing all diseases into causal diseases; it is a quest for cognitive coherence and intelligibility.

As a result, causal disorders represent stipulative decisions created by medicine and adopted by medical grammar. A clear boundary is imposed. The causes of monocriteria disorders are not contingent facts, like scientific causes, but are a priori necessarily true and contain the counterfactual assumption that when the cause is not present, there is no disease. Les désignateurs de maladie dans le cas de maladies causales ne sont donc pas nécessaires mais a priori.

The shift from a descriptive to an etiological and referential taxonomy in the case where it is either microbiological (infectious diseases), nutritional (scurvy) or genetic, reveals the philosopher's stone of medicine, namely the hope of absorbing all diseases into causal diseases; it is a quest for cognitive coherence and intelligibility.

As a result, causal disorders represent stipulative decisions created by medicine and adopted by medical grammar. A clear boundary is imposed. The causes of monocriteria disorders are not contingent facts, like scientific causes, but are a priori necessarily true and contain the counterfactual assumption that when the cause is not present, there is no disease.

In the nosographic framework, groups of sick people can be divided and classified into categories that overlap with the previous subdivision. The identification of Mycobacterium Tuberculosis by Koch led to the decision to change the axis of definition. Brian MacMahon has shown that Cullen's 1785 classification of the sick into four obvious categories—pyrexia, local, neurosis and cachexia—included in each of them patients who would be considered to have tuberculosis today. Diseases with a single criterion are necessarily and a priori causal, because they are the object of a decision that defines them by cause: it is not an empirical cause but a grammatical cause [380, 381].

This means that peptic ulcer is not a causative disease, as H. pylori is not a necessary and sufficient cause. About 90% of duodenal ulcers and 75% of gastric ulcers are associated with *Helicobacter pylori*. It appears to cause damage to the mucosa of the stomach and duodenum by three potential mechanisms: the production of toxins that cause local tissue damage, the induction of a mucosal immune response, and an increase in gastrin levels with increased acid secretion.

The ulcer caused by *H. pylori* is not comparable to the so-called communicable diseases whose cause is grammatical and necessary by stipulation: the presence of Koch's bacillus is necessary for a diagnosis of tuberculosis.

In sum, we should abandon the concept of determinism, so that the final account leaves us with a complex and multifaceted concept of probabilistic causation, to encompass Hans Reichenbach, Patrick Supped, Wesley Salmon, Nancy Cartwright, and Kenneth Schaffner [382]. The lack of predictability is inherent in our situation. The laws of the universe simply say that some events are probable, given other events. Wittgenstein was also interested [383], at various times in his career, in the notion of probability, the probability of a hypothesis or the probability of an event.

The knowledge of the future evolution of a system, guaranteed by the predictive capacity of a theory, is an integral part of the universe described, but the influence of a prediction can never successfully predict everything that covers the system to which it belongs: the self-referential character of the prediction means that it can never predict the future evolution of the system to which it belongs, since, to do so, one would have to wait for the end of its evolution.

In her beautiful book *Medicine and Philosophy*, which is very unphilosophical despite its title, Anne Fagot-Largeault writes a chapter on the history of the development of the concept of cause in medicine until the middle of the twentieth century. There is nothing on the concept of cause in medicine today, nothing on counterfactuals, nothing on supervenience; nothing on the major role of analytical epidemiology in determining causal factors. Nothing either on the philosophical problems raised by causality in science and medicine analyzed by Mackie, J. Pearl, and N. Cartwright.

8.7 Randomized Intervention Trials and Mendelian Randomization

True clinical trials involve the random selection of people from the population, who are then randomly assigned to either treatment or control groups. The type and amount of intervention is dictated by the investigator. There is considerable evidence that LDL (low density lipoproteins), the bad cholesterol, as increased is linked to increased cardiovascular risk, as well as a very low or a very high HDL [384].

On the other hand, natural randomized experiments, Mendelian randomization, could be described as natural experiments, since the type and amount of intervention is dictated by nature, but by the investigator.

For simplicity, let's imagine that there is only one gene and one chromosome that affects serum cholesterol. Let's further imagine that a mutation has occurred such that people who carry it have 10% higher cholesterol and that if both alleles are affected, the cholesterol level is 20% higher. This mutation could be perpetuated and become common in the population.

In the population we will have people with these variants:

(1) High cholesterol variant on both pairs of chromosomes: 10% increase each, giving a total of 20%.
(2) Higher cholesterol variant on one of the chromosomes: 10% increase in cholesterol.
(3) Higher cholesterol variant on neither chromosome pair: normal amount of cholesterol.

The group to which one belongs is determined at conception and at random. Both groups cannot be subject to bias or confounding factors. This makes it possible to directly test the hypothesis that a 10% increase in cholesterol leads to an increased risk of coronary heart disease.

It is then necessary to undertake genetic testing of individuals to find those with the variants described above, and a source of data on the results. Any population sample will do as exposure must precede effect.

The value of Mendelian randomization is that it studies lifetime exposure to low cholesterol and not a few years' exposure to a treatment for high cholesterol.

This method is very interesting for studying weak associations between risk factors and events of interest, particularly in cardiovascular epidemiology.

8.8 The Vicissitudes of 'Risk'

A risk factor is a factor associated with an increased probability of an unfavourable outcome that is potentially but not necessarily a causal factor.

Elodie Giroux has attempted to put some order into a literature that is not always coherent or well founded on the concept of disease risk. She found herself confronted with an inextricable skein to untangle [385]. This term used in ordinary language, as well as in medical language, is extremely ambiguous.

According to one of the two histories of epidemiology [386]: "From the mid-1950s ... Brian MacMahon at Harvard and Abraham Lilienfeld at John Hopkins emphasized the search for individual risk factors as 'exposures' predisposing to chronic disease".

However, as the second history of epidemiology [387] indicates, criticism of the dominance of this model began to proliferate in the 1990s. The limited usefulness of risk factors in recognizing causes at multiple levels and advancing qualitative and quantitative methods began to be seen as a liability.

In the latest edition of his treatise on epidemiology, Rothman has eliminated the term 'risk'. He uses several terms for distinct concepts such as incidence proportion, survival function, regression measure of effect etc. [388].

On the one hand, in epidemiology, risk generally refers to the probability of dying or developing a disease, or its precursors. Risk is often synonymous with incidence [389]. It is also often used in the sense of cause [390].

However, MacMahon and Trichopoulos have pointed out that risks differ from rates in two important respects. First, risks do not have a time dimension as a fundamental component (other than descriptive, indicating the period of an epidemic or an age limit). Second, the reference population is the unaffected population at the beginning of the observation period, as opposed to the average population during the observation period [391].

Patients with high blood pressure or high cholesterol are monitored and put on treatment, but high risks of developing disease seem to be in a grey area between disease and health, and if preventive therapy is effective, they will never get sick. Do risk states challenge the philosophical assumption that disease and health are mutually exclusive? [392].

In saying this, the discourse on risk too often does not avoid the "*risk fallacy that arises from not distinguishing between absolute and relative risk*" [393]. In a large study conducted by the WHO in 11 countries, women who had used contraceptives for at least 5 years had a relative risk of developing cervical cancer of 1.5 compared to non-users [394]. Should this be a concern? The answer is that the difference in life expectancy between users and non-users that would be produced by the increased risk of cervical cancer was 11 days for women aged 20–24 years and 7 days for women aged 30–34 years [395]. This negligible absolute risk contrasts with the relative risk:

$$\text{Relative risk} = \frac{\text{Incidence among those at risk}}{\text{Incidence in the unexposed}}$$

On the other hand, associations are rarely causal, but their analysis is the starting point for understanding causality in epidemiology. The influencing characteristics are called risk factors. However, in epidemiology, risk factors do not necessarily imply that the characteristic has a causal effect, so the term "risk-taker" is sometimes used to emphasize that no causal relationship is involved [396].

Where there is more than a statistical association with a disease, if there is agreement on a causal relationship, the term "*causal factor*" or simply "*cause*" is used.

Risk conditions such as hypertension and hypercholesterolemia have converged with the disease they predict [397]. Using functional magnetic resonance imaging (fMRI), prodromal states of serious neurological or mental illnesses, such as Alzheimer's disease and schizophrenia, are rapidly transformed from risk states to true chronic diseases [398]. Menopause is a risk factor for cardiovascular disease, osteoporosis, type II diabetes and metabolic syndrome. Birth is surprisingly dangerous for modern humans compared to other primates. The pre-ovulatory stage of the menstrual cycle is a significant risk factor for an ACL tear, as experienced by at least one million women each year. Pregnancy is a risk factor. Worldwide, for every 100,000 births in 2017, 211 mothers died. The well-known risk factors for breast cancer are high socio-economic status and being single.

It is to avoid these ambiguities between causes, rates, and risk factors that Brian MacMahon proposed to define epidemiology as the study of the distribution of determinants of disease frequency in human populations.

In conclusion, the different uses of the term 'risk' indicate that it is not an entity, but a family resemblance.

8.9 Meaning and Relativity of Risk

A procedure with a 5% complication rate may seem safe when compared to an alternative with a 25% complication rate. The same 5% complication rate may seem unacceptable when compared to an alternative with a 1% complication rate. When proposing treatment choices to patients, all that matters is the risk/benefit ratio.

Let's imagine a first case. This is a patient with a serious infection. A strong antibiotic can cure the infection, but it can also cause a serious neurological condition that can be fatal. Based on a genetic marker, it is possible to divide patients into a high-risk group, with a 1 in 10 chance of neurological side effects, and a low-risk group, with a 1 in 100 chance of side effects. The patient is in the low-risk group. Should this drug be used for this patient?

Now consider the same case, but with different numbers. Based on a genetic marker, we can divide patients into a low-risk group, which has a 1 in 1000 chance of side effects, and a high-risk group, which has a 1 in 100 chance of side effects. The patient, unfortunately, is in the high-risk group. What about the use of this drug for this patient?

In each of these scenarios, the patient has a 1% risk of serious side effects. It is rational not to care about the patient's risk category. However, by presenting the patient in the "high" and "low" risk groups, the same risk is perceived differently: in the first case, the 1 in 10 risk is presented first, making the 1 in 100 risk seem low. In the second case, the 1 in 1000 risk is presented first, making the 1 in 100 risk seem high [399].

8.10 The Role of Genetics

In the case of what is supposed to be a genetic disease, at least two questions arise. What is the probability that a person will have the disease in question if they have the genetic mutation in question? And what is the probability of a person having the disease in question if they do not have the genetic mutation in question?

Ideal genetic diseases are those in which a particular mutation makes the presence of a disease almost certain and in which the clinical manifestations of that disease are virtually absent in the absence of the genetic mutation. However, in general, a genetic disease means that people who carry the gene are more likely than others to develop the disease.

A distinction must be made between diseases caused by a single gene (monogenetic), those caused by chromosomal abnormalities, and complex diseases associated with variation in many genes as well as environmental variation. In addition, many common conditions (heart disease, diabetes) have a genetic component, so a person's overall genetic make-up is a risk factor for disease, as are environmental factors. Moreover, there is no essence or ontological concept of genetic diseases, as genetic diseases are an illustration of family resemblances.

A *genome-wide association study* (GWAS) is an analysis of many genetic variations in many individuals to study their correlations with phenotypic traits. A GWAS is applied to the entire genome, which allows a higher percentage of variance to be explained for quantitative traits controlled by several genes. In the last 10 years, GWAS technology has transformed genetic research on complex diseases, so that in the first 2 years of its implementation, many loci for several common diseases and traits were identified.

Even with the powerful new GWAS technology, researchers are locating only a small fraction of the genes or, more accurately, loci that explain the genetic influence on traits and diseases. They sometimes refer to this gap between specific genes or loci and the general genetic influence as "missing heritability" or "genetic dark matter" [400].

Basic genomic research has led to major advances in recent years, such as the discovery of microRNAs, long-range promoters, epigenetic factors, and copy number variations. Not surprisingly, the focus on the still unknown genetic mechanisms will largely be on whole-genome resequencing, gene transcription analysis, and genome-wide epigenetics. Rapid advances in biotechnology are making it increasingly feasible to study rare variants in many genes or large genomic regions in larger samples [401].

For example, schizophrenia affects 20 million people worldwide. Research has identified the important role of genes in the disease but isolating individual genes to better understand schizophrenia has proven to be a challenge. It is a very heterogeneous disease, with hundreds or even thousands of genes involved.

Yet it is possible to develop a clinical, phenomenological definition of the syndrome of schizophrenia that would be compatible with the classical concept of Kraepelin and those derived from him, and that would be based on symptoms that are universally encountered and are independent of the cultural and personal biases of the psychiatrist. This suggests that, while schizophrenia is a heterogeneous syndrome, the physiological mechanisms that lead to its clinical profile are probably common and unambiguous.

Because of the ultra-heterogeneity of the disease, it is extremely rare to find a recurrent variant: in a way, the genetics of schizophrenia are so complex that every patient in the world is unique in the genetics that led to their disorder.

8.11 To Conclude

The philosophical problem of causality is at the very heart of medical and epidemiological research. It is quite surprising that the philosophy of medicine has little interest in the two sides of research on this subject, that of epidemiology and that of the philosophy of science [402], which are the subject of a considerable number of publications that leave little trace in the philosophy of medicine [403].

Chapter 9
Medical Explanation

We have no right to establish any kind of theory... We must discard all explanation and put only description in its place.
Wittgenstein [404]

Abstract Medical explanation may consist in hierarchical research, reduction, supervenience, inference to the best explanation. The degree of inductive liability of an argument is the probability that its conclusion is true, given that its premises are true (the Bayes theorem). Medicine moves form realism to instrumentalism and to praxeology. Traditional Cartesianism is leading to the philosophy of neuroscience. Neo-Darwinism leads to adaptationism and the Panglossian Fallacy.

Keywords Explanation · Induction · Abduction · Reduction · Supervenience · Essence & family resemblances · Realism vs instrumentalism · Neurosciences · Adaptationism · The Panglossian fallacy

How do we differentiate causality from explanation?

James Lovelock writes: "As Newton discovered long ago, logical thinking does not work with dynamic systems, things can change over time. Quite simply, you can't explain the workings of anything living by cause-and-effect logic" [405].

In everyday language and even in philosophical thinking, causality is often not differentiated from explanation, whereas causality comes first in medical thinking.

The fact that *Helicobacter pylori* is the main determinant of gastric ulcer was known for more than 20 years before it was accepted by the medical community [406]. This causal relationship was initially rejected because it seemed impossible that certain bacteria could attack the stomach wall in its acidic and hostile environment. Criticism of the explanation delayed the acceptance of a specific causal factor.

In fact, in most analytical epidemiological studies, it is the causal relationships that are at stake, not the explanatory theories: we knew that cigarette smoking increases the likelihood of lung cancer before we knew the type of carcinogens in tobacco smoke and their carcinogenic role. Thus, the evidence for a causal relationship between smoking and lung cancer has been unequivocal for several decades,

L. Karhausen, *The Fragility of Philosophy of Medicine*, Philosophy and Medicine 147, https://doi.org/10.1007/978-3-031-41633-0_9

even if the how's and whys of this relationship have long remained incomplete. In other words, causal statements tell us that A gives rise to B, while scientific explanatory theories and laws tell us why A leads to B. The study of a causal effect does not require knowledge of its mechanism.

Other examples. Aspirin was used as a painkiller a century before the effect of prostaglandins was discovered, and lithium was used to treat bipolar syndrome long before its mechanism of action on the brain was known.

On the one hand, to cause something is to produce something, to provoke something. On the other hand, scientific knowledge allows us to explain why things happen as they do. There is having that and knowing how.

For Donald Davidson [407] and Elizabeth Anscombe [408], causality is an extensional relation that is established between events, while explanation is an intensional relation that is established between events within a description. Causal connections in nature behave extensionally since a cause is external to its effect, and its effect is its extension, namely the object to which it refers. In contrast, explanatory relations, and the content of explanations, being linguistic, behave intensionally.

In medicine, we speak metaphorically of the mechanism of a disease when we refer to its pathogenesis and explanatory theories. Causes contribute to the existence of their effects, while explanation, i.e., pathogenesis or mechanism, refers to the way in which a given causal relationship functions and requires process complexes.

The debate on so-called black box epidemiology illustrates this confusion. A black box is explained only in terms of inputs and outputs; the internal mechanism that converts inputs into outputs is obscured. According to David Hume, it is not necessary to know the inner workings of a black box to establish the causal relationship between input and output. We knew why the apple fell on Newton's nose, even though gravitation was not yet fully understood. In other words, we can have evidence of causality in the absence of a full explanation [409].

An *explanandum*, i.e., what needs to be explained, for example a disease, describes a change. Causes and effects are the temporal ends of changes. An explanation therefore consists of filling in the gaps between them and explaining the intermediate steps or the course of events that lie between the temporal starting and ending points of a change. It follows that the gaps are like blanks in an already prepared conditional expectation framework [410]. In the meantime, it is not essential to know this range of events to resolve questions of causality. It is usually knowledge of the latter that can enable us to launch a prevention programme despite our ignorance of the former.

It is a very popular idea that medicine is both an art and a science, which goes hand in hand with the idea that it is both objective and subjective, and that it combines both facts and values. However, Thomas Cunningham, in a brilliant analysis, rejects a dualist epistemology of medicine. It is better to see medicine as an integrative science aiming at a multilevel explanation in the service of the patient's health, rather than as a science on the one hand and an art on the other [411].

9.1 Induction and Abduction: Inference Towards the Best Explanation

In contrast to the strict coverage law explanation based on deductive inferences, epidemiological reasoning turns out to be inductive rather than deductive. From true premises that have some empirical content, it supports a conclusion, not by showing that it is true, but simply that it is reasonably probable.

Hypothetico-deductive and inductive-statistical models represent a low-risk strategy in that they avoid the danger of immediate false beliefs. However, there is a price to pay for such security. A strategy that is likely to provide useful truths accepts a greater risk that some results may sometimes be wrong. The price for accepting the epistemic risk, namely the possibility of some false beliefs, should be a greater chance of obtaining useful true beliefs.

The general idea proposed by Peter Lipton is that a hypothesis gains inductive support if, added to our stock of previously accepted beliefs, it allows us to explain something we observe or believe, if no competing explanation works nearly as well. A hypothesis provides the best explanation when it is more explanatory, broader, more modest, more powerful, more falsifiable, and generally more conservative than any competing hypothesis. Such a strategy is the best explanation inference.

One of the most common forms of inductive argument is a concept formulated by Gilbert Harman [412], but it is sometimes also called *abduction*, a term introduced by Charles Sanders Pierce (1839–1914). Gilbert Harman writes: "*Inference to the best explanation*" roughly corresponds to what others have called "abduction", "hypothesis method", "hypothetical inference", "method of elimination", "eliminative induction" and "theoretical inference".

In everyday problems, we usually adopt the solution that best explains them. In the hypothetical-deductive method, we try to make sense of a hypothesis by deducing it from well-established premises. With inference to the best explanation, we reason in the opposite direction, since we derive the explanation from the observation instead of deriving an observation from its explanation.

Philosophy may be needed to correct errors in medical reasoning. The brilliant treatise *Modern Epidemiology* [413], now in its fourth edition, repeats in each successive edition the same error of rejecting inductivism based on a certain reading of Karl Popper, in ignorance of the fact that the philosophy of science is evolving, as is epidemiology.

The logic of abduction, i.e., inference to the best explanation, is a major concern in science. Most elements of reasoning in science and medicine are achieved by arguing towards the best explanation. The treatment of mental illness, long dominated by psychoanalysis, has been transformed by inductive explanation with pharmacological research such as the discovery of chlorpromazine, with electroconvulsive therapy and with cognitive psychotherapy.

Yet medical scientists may continue to use a theory in the face of counterevidence, which sometimes perpetuates errors. Until the early twentieth century, doctors used to reduce high fevers by inducing diarrhea with a purgative combined with bloodletting, thus depriving patients of valuable fluids and electrolytes. In 1927, a discussion presented by W.G. Spencer on bloodletting, its past and present was held at the Royal Society of Medicine, a century after the groundbreaking publication by Pierre-Charles-Alexandre-Louis (1787–1872) which showed not only that bloodletting was ineffective but also that it increased mortality.

Furthermore, during the twentieth century, scientists and statisticians developed methods to manage epistemic risks and quantify uncertainty and evidence, focusing mainly on the use of a statistical significance level of p 0.05 and the avoidance of Type I error. Jerzy Neyman and Egon Pearson provided a method for making a choice between hypotheses. They described two types of error: Type I error, or false positive, and Type II error, or false negative. In Type I error, the experimenter rejects the null hypothesis of no treatment differences, when it is in fact true. In the Type II error, the experimenter does not reject the null hypothesis when it is false.

The reduction in Type I errors can only be achieved at the cost of an increase in Type II errors. This means that reducing the number of false positives in the long run will increase the number of false negatives.

Furthermore, in pathophysiological studies and epidemiological investigations, one is dealing with complex multifactorial processes involving small or weak associations and the more variables one includes in the analysis, the less plausible the null hypothesis.

In other words, the increasing sophistication of our methodological and statistical tools allows medical scientists to detect more subtle phenomena, thus increasing the risk of erroneous results.

Finally, it is necessary to determine what degree of epistemic risk is acceptable, as externalities, i.e., non-scientific constraints, must be considered when setting the standard of proof. Mark Parascandola, in his historical report on epistemic risk, has shown how, in the twentieth century, scientists and philosophers developed methods in public health and medicine to manage epistemic risk and quantify the degrees of uncertainty and evidential support [414].

9.2 Rational Choice Maximizes Utility

The degree of inductive reliability of an argument is the probability that its conclusion is true given that its premises are true. It is possible to formulate the problem of induction in terms of degrees of certainty using Bayes' theorem.

First, in Bayes' theorem, the initial probability distribution embodies the plausibility of the hypotheses of a research project. The process of confirming a hypothesis H starts with an initial probability; new data from the experiment E then confirms this hypothesis if it increases the initial probability: $P(H/E) > P(H)$; it negates this hypothesis if it decreases the initial probability: $P(H/E) < P(H.)$

Second, the conditional probability, i.e., the probability of a hypothesis H, given empirical evidence E is equal to the joint probabilities of hypothesis H and evidence E, divided by evidence E:

(1) $\frac{P\ (H\&E)}{P(E)}$

Finally, Bayes' theorem allows us to revise our beliefs in the light of experience, and provides a basis for a theory of inductive experience:

(2) $\frac{P\ (H/E) = P\ (E/H)\ P\ (H)}{P(E)}$

In Bayes' theorem, the subjectivity lies in the initial probability, while the posterior probability obeys the probability axioms. Subjective probability is a very vague notion. However, it is shown that this does not matter, because this subjectivity decreases and eventually disappears in the face of successive data from the experiment.

The Bayesian approach is used to obtain and interpret diagnostic information [415], to model causality [416], to compare or contrast randomized controlled trials with Bayesian methods [417]. Bayesian methods are used in clinical trials and by the pharmaceutical industry, but so far have not been of much use in medical practice.

Furthermore, Nancy Cartwright has always been very skeptical of the Bayesian method. "Addiction may be due to causation," writes Nancy Cartwright. But there are many other reasons for it. In her Social Science Methods course, she advises, "If you see a probabilistic dependence and are inclined to infer causation, think carefully about all the other possible reasons why the dependence might occur and eliminate them one by one. And when you have finished, remember that your conclusion is no more certain than your belief that you have really eliminated all possible alternatives" [418].

9.3 Medical Explanation

Explanation answers the question "Why?" and allows us to understand: sometimes it gives us the ability to control and predict and sometimes it explains by saying what something is made of.

Wittgenstein suggests that "*We want to establish an order in our knowledge of the use of language; an order for a particular purpose; an order among many possible ones; not the Order*" [419].

The covering law model, namely the *hypothetico-deductive model*, which attempts to identify general laws, does not apply to medicine, as there are no laws of nature as such in biology. The explanations proposed by the inductive-statistical model are more fruitful. The inference to the best explanation is in the opposite direction, since one derives the explanation from the observation instead of deriving an observation from its explanation.

Synoptically, medical explanation evolves along two axes, which are complementary and interlocking, but which are, in metaphorical language, perpendicular to each other: the mechanistic biomedical axis, which follows "vertically" from a reductionist point of view, and the epidemiological approach, which deals with the causal horizon and its stochastic uncertainties.

The explanation contrasts with a conventional-normative and counterfactual context. All diseases reveal a disruption of certain counterfactual processes considered ‘normal’ and explanation in medicine contrasts with a conventional-normative and counterfactual context.

In sum, knowledge of causes is possible without a satisfactory understanding of what is involved in causation. A mechanism is a local biological process, a causal pathway from cause to effect [420].

9.4 Reduction

A first method on which biomedical research is based is that of reduction [421].

The human being is a multilevel structure, and it is very common to differentiate several levels of biological organization: physical microparticles, certain chemical compounds, cells, tissues, organs, organ systems, the organism. The different levels seem to express different properties, but not in isolation, with a higher level needing the support of lower levels. The properties of higher levels seem to emerge from the properties of lower levels; they tend to be more complicated and complex in nature. Biological reductionism has been successful in modern medicine.

To reduce a concept is to define it in relation to others and thus to eliminate it from the list of basic entities in the field under consideration. Reductionists in medicine, for example, argue that diseases can be reduced to the analysis of pathological findings. The reduction is towards less complexity, simpler phenomena, and fewer models. It has a reverse process, that of integration, which involves moving to a complex causal structure of interactions, to larger scales or higher levels, and to proceed between several overlapping models.

Reduction is a widely used and useful research tool both methodologically and conceptually. Methodologically, it allows a disease to be viewed in terms of less complex sub-mechanisms, each of which can potentially be the subject of an independent intervention.

This style of vertical explanation asserts that the best explanatory strategy is to attempt to explain a disease process, or clinical disease, in terms of entities at lower levels: it moves down the hierarchical ladder, and the explanation ends when it reaches the level of normal states or processes. Physiopathological research is thus based on a hierarchical explanatory model, what Nancy Cartwright calls “*downward reduction*”: [422] it assumes a multilevel causal/mechanical explanation that claims to explain complex medical phenomena in terms of simpler, more fundamental characteristics. The logic of this model is based on the premise that clinical facts are what require explanation, as all medical negativities, abnormal and pathological events or processes originate exclusively at the clinical level.

Explanation by mechanistic biomedical research, namely the vertical style of explanation, assumes that there is a hierarchy of different levels of phenomenal reality. It assumes a multi-level causal/mechanical explanation that claims to explain complex medical phenomena in terms of simpler, more fundamental characteristics. The nomological structure of this model is based on the premise that clinical facts are essential, as all medical negativities, abnormal and pathological events or processes originate exclusively at the clinical level. Methodological reductionism claims that the best explanatory strategy is to attempt an explanation in terms of lower-level entities. Mechanistic biomedical research moves down the hierarchical ladder, and the explanation stops when it reaches the level of normal states or processes.

Reduction can therefore help researchers to isolate the early causal stages of these diseases and to isolate the main factors of a disease in a population where there may be a wide variety of causes, and a few common causes or causal pathways in most cases. Reduction is also useful for guiding interventions in a causal chain through prevention or treatment. Conceptually, reduction can help to understand how different models of the same or closely related phenomena relate to each other, so that we can use these distinct models in appropriate circumstances.

9.5 Supervenience

A second form of explanation is that of supervenience [423]. Things of type A are supererogatory to things of type B, when the presence or absence of things of type A is completely determined by the presence or absence of things of type B; there can be no difference in type A without a difference in type B, although there can be differences in B without differences in A. A clear example of the supervenience of clinical over biochemical data: clinical manifestations have medical properties by virtue of their biochemical properties, and there can be no clinical difference without a biochemical difference.

We need such a kind of dependency relationship that is not reductive, namely a necessary dependent variation or covariation that strives to be either causal, logical, emergent, or probabilistic. An example of the supervenience of the clinical over the physicochemical: patients have diabetes (A) by virtue of biochemical abnormalities (B), and there can be no diabetes (A) without such biochemical abnormalities (B) [424].

Supervenience is characterized by temporal symmetry (as opposed to temporal asymmetry in the case of causality) and spatial direction. Supervenience properties determine supervenience properties, but the latter are not reducible to the former.

Supervenience is distinct from reduction: when, to be a process of kind A, nothing other than a process of kind B is required. Those who defend the supervenience of the mental over the physical argue that mental categories are neither identical nor reducible to physical categories. Thus, there is no mental difference without a physical difference, but mental categories are not equivalent to physical categories.

Contrary to Kenneth Schaffner's assertion that molecular biology and the Watson-Crick model have reduced the laws of classical genetics to physical and chemical laws, so that "gene sequences of DNA", David Hull pointed out that these relationships are "*many-many*" relationships and not "*one-one*" or "*many-one*" relationships as Schaffner assumes [425]; because phenomena characterized by a single predicate can be reproduced by several types of molecular mechanism and conversely, the same type of molecular mechanism can produce phenomena characterized by different predicate terms [426]. Hull [427] insisted "on the necessary one-to-one or many-to-one relationships that lead from molecular predicate terms to Mendelian predicate terms", to account for this divergence and to meet the intuition or need to speak of a reduction from classical to molecular genetics. Alexander Rosenberg adopted the notion of supervenience to describe the relationship between classical and molecular genetics [428].

9.6 The Limits of Explanation

Wittgenstein, like Quine, rejected reductionism. "How can I now understand the sentence if the analysis is to show me just what I understand" [429].

According to Wittgenstein, the laws of nature determine how scientific propositions can be derived from 'axioms', and thus what form specific generalizations and descriptions can take. But natural laws do not describe the necessities of the world since the only necessity is logical. Indeed, they do not provide an explanation of why things happen as they do. In the absence of physical necessities, what happens in the world is raw contingency; it cannot be explained by reference to the operation of inviolable natural laws any more than it can be explained by invoking fate.

In contrast, the law of induction expresses the empirical proposition that our forms of description will continue to adapt to future events in the same way as they have done in the past [430]. In the context of a chosen model, we proceed by induction, which means that we opt for the simplest law that corresponds to our experience. This law is then used as a basis for prediction and prevention. However, there is no logical justification for this procedure, so that the principles underlying scientific theories or models are conventions.

Moreover, since, unlike physics, there are no laws in biology or medicine, the models are not general but particular.

Wittgenstein scattered remarks that prefigured Kuhn's notion [431] of a scientific paradigm and that inform the way a scientific theory responds to evidence. The nature of medical explanation generally corresponds to what he called forms of representation (*Form der Darstellung*), i.e., how we see things [432]. The apparent essence of reality is only a shadow of the grammar, and the grammar represents our form of representation. A form of representation determines the meaning of key scientific expressions. But it does not just label things, it provides a way of making sense of experience, making predictions, and thus informing complex scientific practices. The changes in our forms of representation are far from trivial in their motives and consequences: they do not simply mean a change of name, but a new way of theorizing the world.

Wittgenstein writes: "*Hypotheses such as 'invisible masses', 'unconscious mental events' are standards of expression. They enter language to enable us to say that there must be causes... We believe that we are dealing with an a priori natural law, whereas we are dealing with an expressive norm that we ourselves have set... The statement that there must be a cause shows that we have a rule of language. The question whether all speeds can be explained by the hypothesis of invisible masses is a question of mathematics, or of grammar, and is not to be settled by experience*" [433].

For Nancy Cartwright the laws of nature are empirically false, which is in line with Wittgenstein's view that they are merely grammatical.

Wittgenstein observes: "*In every language there is a bridge between the sign and its application. No one can do it for us; we must bridge that gap ourselves. No explanation ever saves the leap, for any further explanation will itself require a leap.*"

Wittgenstein's thinking here is very close to Lewis Carroll's parable in "*What the Turtle Says to Achilles*". The tortoise grants Achilles premises from which a certain conclusion follows but refuses to grant the conclusion. When Achilles points out that if the premises are true, the conclusion must also be true, the tortoise seems to accept Achilles' assertion, adding it to his set of premises, but still refuses the conclusion. And each time Achilles insists that if the most recent expanded premises are true, the conclusion must be true as well, the tortoise responds by expanding its set of premises again to incorporate Achilles' latest insistence (without drawing the conclusion).

The turtle is asking for a self-executing rule, one that will bridge the gap between the premises and the conclusion on its own without it having to do anything. And of course, each new insistence by Achilles, interpreted as a new premise, simply hangs in the air with what it interprets, and does not bring the conclusion any closer.

Achilles would do well to respond to the tortoise with a remark from Wittgenstein: "*I am not trying to make you believe something you do not believe, but to make you do something you will not do* [434]. Not at all pile of premises can replace the action of drawing the conclusion. Following a rule is like an act of decision because our action when we follow a rule is free from logical determination by something outside it: we blindly obey the rule.

9.7 Essence or Family Resemblance

The meaning of a word such as 'disease', 'health', is usually associated with the 'thing' to which it refers. And this raises an interesting question: is there ever anything central or common to ordinary word usages?

John Locke's idea of the true essences of words was revived by Hilary Putnam and by Kripke. When it was found that some substances that were once called 'gold' because they met superficial criteria of similarity, had a different atomic structure from gold, it was not concluded that gold does not always have the atomic number 79, but that this is what distinguished real gold from other similar substances. If a word has one or two or more characteristics that cannot be taken away, it is simply because of the way we are culturally and intellectually acclimatized in our present habits.

The meaning of a word is its usage, its use in language. Usage determines the meaning of a word by giving it ordinary or extended, i.e., fluctuating, meanings [435].

Wittgenstein writes: "*In science it is usual to make phenomena that allow for precise measurement in the definition of the criteria of an expression; and one is then inclined to think that now the correct meaning has been found. Innumerable confusions have thus arisen. There are degrees of pleasure, but it is foolish to speak of a measure of pleasure. It is true that in some cases a measurable phenomenon occupies the place previously occupied by a non-measurable phenomenon. Then the word for this place changes its meaning, and its former meaning has become obsolete. We are appeased by the fact that the first concept is the more exact, the other the more inaccurate, and we do not notice that here, in each case a different relation is in question between the concept of "exact" and "inaccurate": this is the old mistake of not dealing with particular cases*" [436].

Wittgenstein is opposed, on the one hand, to the idea that there is something essential to the instances of a concept in virtue of which they are instances of that concept; on the other hand, he is opposed to the idea that any mental process is necessary to mediate between language and the world. These two ideas are intimately linked in Wittgenstein's thinking.

But, in his view, what is in a certain sense simplifying is the idea that all instances of a concept must have something in common. The question is not whether a particular definition can be criticized, but whether the very attempt to fix a set of essential characteristics—necessary and sufficient—is misguided.

If we consider the wide variety of concepts for which appropriate characteristics can be given, we find that most of them are related to each other by *a network of overlapping and intersecting similarities: sometimes global similarities, sometimes similarities of detail*, and not by a characteristic or set of characteristics that all instances have in common. Wittgenstein's concern is not to show that there could not be such a concept, but simply that a concept need not be as such.

There is no better expression to characterize these similarities than *'family resemblances'*, because the various similarities between members of a family: height, features, eye colour, gait, temperament, etc., overlap and intersect in the same way.

9.8 Realism, Instrumentalism and Praxiology

The most powerful insight motivating realism is an old idea, commonly referred to in recent discussions as the 'non-miracle argument', after Hilary Putnam's well-known claim that realism "*is the only philosophy that does not make the success of science a miracle*". The argument begins with the widely accepted premise that our best theories are extraordinarily successful: they facilitate predictions, retrodictions and empirical explanations of the objects of scientific investigation, often marked by stunning precision and complex causal manipulations of the phenomena under discussion. How do we explain this success?

The explanation is that our best theories are true (or approximately true, or correctly describe a world of mind-independent entities, laws, etc.). Indeed, if these theories were far from the truth, the fact that they perform so well would be miraculous. And if, however, one has a choice between a direct explanation of success and a miraculous explanation, one should prefer the non-miraculous explanation, namely that our best theories are approximately true [437].

Scientific realism admits that there are entities that exist in this world independently of our minds. It asserts that scientific or medical theories are about things that are real, like the familiar objects around us. He argues that some theories are literally and objectively true and others literally and objectively false. Moreover, a theory can be wrong even if it was a very good instrument for prediction and intervention. Until 1982, i.e., before the link with *H. pylori* was identified, gastric ulcers were successfully treated with antacids and drugs that block acid production.

Realism involves the conjunction of two theses: (1) an independence thesis: our judgments answer for their truth to a world that exists independently of them or their consciousness; (2) a knowledge thesis: overall, we can know which of these judgments are true.

Realism is opposed to instrumentalism, which claims that scientific theories are merely devices for making predictions and that the objects mentioned in the theory may only be useful myths. It is what Aristotle called a *technè*. We want to know which therapy, which drug is effective against which diseases. The truth of a medical doctrine is not in itself practically relevant: all that matters in medical care is the truth of its observable consequences. Knowing only the molecular processes of a disease will not predict what the disease looks like. According to instrumentalism, a scientific theory should be seen as an instrument to control events, but not necessarily to generate reliable and true predictions or to describe the world accurately.

There is a distinction to be made between observable and unobservable entities. Medical knowledge must then be understood as a tool. We do not need to assume that the terms of the theory—for example, the concepts of function or disease category—refer to anything: these words do not need to bear any deep resemblance to the theory's description of them, if it works.

Clinicians believe in scientific realism and the foundation of scientific knowledge. But they also consider a scientific theory as a *technè,* an instrument to produce new control techniques: this second position reflects *pragmatic allegiances*. Realism tends to privilege one form of knowledge as 'true', whereas for pragmatists, knowledge is not a representation of reality or a 'mirror of nature', but a tool for action. Instead of asking: "Does this knowledge accurately reflect the underlying reality?", the question becomes: "Does this knowledge serve our purposes?" This approach rejects or dismisses large amounts of empirical research, since only humanly manipulable determinants or causes are the appropriate focus. Knowledge of the genome is of great theoretical interest, but at present it still corresponds to few manipulable interventions.

Let us recall that Nancy Cartwright develops a rather convincing argument that science in general is a *technè*, and not, as is customary, an *episteme* [438].

The principle of pragmatism, which emphasizes method over doctrine, instrumentalism over realism, practicality over principle, resembles a "bottom-up", inductive or abductive theory of truth. Scientific realism, a "top-down" procedure, which deduces general propositions to arrive at concrete conclusions about particular cases, is too far removed from the workings of clinical or public health context and experience, even if it remains essential for physiopathological research. Medical nosology is pragmatic. Our aim is to predict and, if possible, successfully manipulate the world without concern for metaphysics, or whether the constructs we develop to help us do so are 'real' or not.

For example, Kendell and Jablensky make a clear distinction between diagnostic validity and diagnostic utility. They write: "*We propose that a diagnostic rubric can be said to have utility if it provides non-trivial information about prognosis and likely treatment outcomes, and/or verifiable propositions about biological and social correlates...*" [439].

Finally, knowledge translation refers to all activities related to the dissemination and transfer of research from the laboratory, research journals and academic conferences to people and organizations that can make practical use of it. Knowledge transfer is very context sensitive. Knowledge to action illustrates the relative roles of realism and instrumentalism in health care. "*There is a distinction to be made between doing the right thing [such as adhering to EBM (evidence-based medicine) guidelines*," writes Peter Drucker, "*and doing the thing (such as adopting interventions and treatments) in light of the needs and context of that person*" [440].

Evidence-Based Medicine (EBM) was introduced in 1992 as a new approach to teaching the practice of medicine, claiming to represent a paradigm shift from an emphasis on intuition, unsystematic clinical experience, and pathophysiological reasoning as sufficient bases for clinical decision-making to an emphasis on the review of evidence from clinical research. This definition has evolved over time. The 2005 definition states that evidence-based medicine requires the integration of the best research evidence with clinical expertise and the unique values and circumstances of the patient.

By attributing the term "pathological" to suffering, medical language places itself here in a descriptive relationship external to biological and clinical reality. As scientists, doctors are not part of the reality in question.

But the situation is different when clinicians make an epistemic about-face, i.e., hen physiology or whatever is counterfactually called "normal" becomes the basis for comparison. With this second position, our experience, the biologist's experience of the world, remains intact; there is no difference between the biological facts before and after this inversion, and since no experience can distinguish between these two points of view, the difference between them is therefore outside experience and is grammatical.

What differentiates them is that in the second position, the medical gaze is constrained by normality in whose counterfactual shadow the whole field of medical research, clinical medicine, and public health, will unfold and bear fruit. This means that clinical medicine, as practical knowledge, deals with contrasts and comparisons between normal and abnormal characteristics and the attraction of normal and physiological counterfactual structures and processes.

Medical language then becomes a kind of complex box of tools or language acts to be used in clinical or public health contexts, which are performative. Doctors and their language now belong to the world they study and try to modulate. They are no longer practicing a natural science and are no longer external observers but participating observers. Medical language is now part of, and internal to, the world it describes [441]. Medical knowledge not only tells us what is happening in the biological world, but also how it should be and what goals we should achieve. Descriptive words recede as language becomes performative and prescriptive, while propositional knowledge gives way to practical knowledge. Medical statements and decisions become a matter of correct or incorrect use, rather than a matter of truth or falsity.

Evidence-based medicine is an ambitious project that consists of applying the methods of clinical epidemiology to the clinical problems that Maël Lemoine has outlined [442].

The distinction of levels of evidence leads to a strict hierarchy: meta-analyses of randomized clinical trials, "observational" studies on real populations, evidence from pathophysiology, and finally those based on expert opinion.

This is a paradigm shift designed to provide a sound scientific basis for medicine. The validity of this paradigm depends on reliable data from clinical trials, most of which are conducted by the pharmaceutical industry and reported in the name of high-level academics.

However, the pharmaceutical industry is accountable to its shareholders, so scientific progress has been thwarted because the industry suppresses negative trial results, fails to report adverse events, and does not share raw data with the academic research community. Patients are dying because of the negative impact of commercial interests.

As a result, academic departments become instruments of industry by controlling the research agenda and writing articles in medical journals, so that academics become agents for the promotion of commercial products.

Industry critics face rejection from journals, legal threats, and potential destruction of their careers. The preservation of institutions designed to foster scientific objectivity (e.g., public laboratories, independent journals, and congresses) is entirely at the mercy of political and commercial power: vested interests will always trump rationality of evidence. Regulators themselves receive funding from industry and use industry-funded and industry-conducted trials to approve drugs, without seeing the raw data in most cases.

What confidence can we have in a system in which pharmaceutical companies are both customers and regulators, rather than having their products tested by independent experts under a public regulatory system? [443].

9.9 Neuroscience and Philosophy

The leading figures of the first two generations of modern brain neuroscientists were basically Cartesian, i.e. that life consists of two parts: a mental and a physical part (Paul and Patricia Churchland, Stephen Stich and Francis Crick); these authors distinguished the mind from the brain and assigned psychological attributes to the mind.

The third generation of neuroscientists (Antonio Damasio, J.P. Frisby, Colin Blakemore, Gerald Edelman, David Marr) rejected dualism and assigned psychological attributes not to the mind, but to the brain or parts of the brain. Most anti-Cartesians think that by rejecting mind/body dualism, they must accept a kind of behaviourism, or a kind of crude materialism.

In contrast, Wittgenstein shows that if we examine the 'deep grammar' of this vocabulary, we do not find two distinct phenomena, one mental and one physical. When we say things like: *'He has been moaning and suffering for two hours'*, we do not feel that we have mixed up the categories, by saying that physical moaning is not to be associated with mental pain.

The question we face is a philosophical one, not a scientific one. It is not possible to investigate experimentally whether or not brains think, believe, guess, reason, etc., until we know what this means for a brain, i.e. until we clarify the meaning of these expressions and what can be considered as brain action and what is the meaning of the statements that attribute these attributes to the brain.

Wittgenstein rejects vulgar reductionism [444], and writes: "*Now, does this mean that it is absurd to speak of a place where thought takes place? ...But if we say, 'Thought takes place in our heads', what is the meaning of this locution...? I imagine that it is that certain physiological processes correspond to our thoughts in such a way that, if we know the correspondence, we can discover the thoughts by observing these processes. But in what sense can we say that physiological processes correspond to thoughts, and in what sense can we say that we access thoughts by observing the brain?*".

Glannon rejects Changeux's reductionist claim that the "final" explanation of human behaviour will come from the study of neurons alone. If it is true that neuronal activity cannot explain human consciousness, human consciousness is unthinkable without neuronal activity. The emergence of the mind from the brain cannot be explained entirely in terms of brain function, because, as emergent, the mind consists of qualitatively new properties that are not represented by the physical properties of the brain [445].

This application of psychological predicates to the brain makes no sense. It is not that brains do not think, decide, see, hear, and answer questions, but it makes no sense to attribute these predicates or their negations to the brain. The brain is not a logically appropriate subject for psychological predicates [446]. Moreover, brain states and processes are not intentional, i.e., they are not directed towards someone or something; they are not defined by the fact that they are about something [447].

The difficulty is whether a first-person, subjective phenomenology of experience can be captured by a third-person, physical, objective explanation of brain structure and function alone.

The theory most often invoked to solve this problem is supervenience, which holds that there is a unidirectional dependence of higher-level mental properties on lower-level physical properties. Each mental property has a physical basis in the brain that guarantees its instantiation. However, supervenience does not recognize that there is a two-way dependency relationship between mind and brain and between brain and mind. Moreover, it is too general a theory to explain the complexity of the emergence of mental properties and physical states embedded in the brain.

One could argue that mental states are supervenient to widely distributed neural networks. But this would not recognize the interdependence of the brain and mind and the influence of the environment on the brain-mind relationship. The mind-body problem requires a tripartite structure that includes the relationships between the brain, the body, and the external environment.

Gilbert Ryle has proposed that we avoid abstract questions such as "What kind of thing is a mind?" and instead examine how we use words like "mind", "mental", etc. in ordinary language. If we do this, we will conclude that 'mind' is not the name of a thing, but a way of classifying a wide variety of human activities and other dispositions.

Incidentally, the neuroscientist establishes normal brain function based on observed abnormalities. The external evaluation tests that result from observation have always provided a negative induction, i.e., from the clinical finding of dysfunction. These pathologies are always expressed in a negative way, such as aphasia, amnesia, blindness, etc. Brain imaging reveals the impact of long-term depression.

Furthermore, biomarkers are becoming increasingly important in psychiatry.

A recent study by the UMC-C-Vrije Universiteit in the Netherlands, presented in September 2021 at the 33rd Congress of the European College of Neuropsychopharmacology (ECNP), showed that a subtype of depression is associated with several blood biomarkers.

Similarly, Dr Alexander B. Niculescu III, MD, PhD, professor of psychiatry and medical neuroscience at Indiana University School of Medicine in Indianapolis, and colleagues have identified 13 RNA markers from the basis of a blood test that can not only diagnose depression, but also predict who will develop bipolar disorder, who is likely to become ill enough to require hospital treatment in the future, and which medications are most likely to be effective in particular cases [448].

Alternatively, *autoimmunity* may also play a role in psychiatric disorders. Certain classes of cytokines, and possibly autoantibodies, may have a negative effect on cognition, mood, and volition. Depression, anorexia nervosa and bulimia have been associated with these immune mechanisms. Infectious agents such as viruses and psychological stress can activate the immune system and cause the release of cytokines. Cytokines are secreted by lymphoid cells and are immunomodulatory in the sense that they amplify some immune responses and inhibit others.

Finally, some researchers are working on the production of neurochemicals from the microbiome, i.e., from the 100 trillion micro-organisms that live mainly in the human gut. They have been shown to play a crucial role in gut-brain communication by influencing neural, immune, and endocrine pathways.

In other words, much brain activity is affected by what happens elsewhere in the body. This underlines the fact that mental disorders must be considered from a holistic body perspective where regulatory physiological systems such as immunity and lipid metabolism are involved. Is depression then a brain dysfunction, a disorder of the mind, or a disease that affects the whole person. Who we are as people is determined by the nature and content of our mental states.

The most important conclusion is that mental disorders cannot be fully or satisfactorily explained by a simple dysfunction of the brain. In other words, they are not disorders of the brain, but disorders in the brain [449].

Mereology is the logic of part/whole relations. Psychological predicates apply only to human beings or other animals; they cannot be intelligibly applied to their parts, such as the brain, for this would be to commit the mereological fallacy [450].

I would conclude, with Walter Glannon, professor at the University of Calgary in Canada, that psychiatric disorders are, in a sense, not mental illnesses, that they are neither diseases of the mind nor diseases of the body, but diseases of the person [451].

Adaptationism and the Panglossian fallacy

"*Why do parasites harm their hosts*?" asks Pierre Olivier Méthot. One is tempted to ask him, "*Why not?*" or again, "*Most parasites do not harm their hosts and are sometimes useful to them.*" In an article published in 2013, Gomez showed that parasites can organize ecosystems, and that often a parasite protects its host from another more harmful parasite [452].

But why this question? This question raises another: what are the implicit premises of this question? What is the tacit intention behind this request?

Evolutionary medicine has developed rapidly over the last two or three decades [453]. The very concept of evolutionary medicine [454] as a purely biological discipline seems misplaced, as evolutionary explanations in medicine are highly speculative and have little or no empirical verification [455]. They assume that evolution is always progressive [456], which Broadbent calls the *adaptationist fallacy* [457].

Pierre-Olivier Méthot presented a summary of evolutionary explanations in medicine [458]. He compares the retrospective ultimate explanation with prospective predictive models. Most of his chapter covers the history of evolutionary medicine. In addition to several medical fallacies such as the adaptive value of fever [459] and the neglect of non-Darwinian explanations, the field of evolutionary medicine offers little more than speculative hypotheses about our ancestral past; it illustrates the naturalistic fallacy that the healthy functioning of the individual cannot be deduced from its evolutionary history, as Cournoyea's clarification indicates [460]. Moreover, this approach often confuses two distinct concepts: evolution and selection.

This Panglossian fallacy has its roots in the teleological myth that evolution is always progressive because natural selection eliminates the unfit. Demography and epidemiology contradict this view, showing that plagues and wars have eliminated entire well-adapted peoples, along with their unique genomes [461].

For example, the plague that killed half the population of the Byzantine Empire between 541 and the eighth century may have opened the doors to the expansion of Islam. Biology cannot explain any of the biosocial processes that have altered the course of history, if only because it focuses on biotic processes in individuals, not on social processes.

Why do we get sick? Evolutionary medicine believes it will answer this question because, according to Nesse and Stearns, "it will transform the way patients and doctors view disease" [462]. Pierre-Olivier Méthot sought to define disease from a Darwinian perspective [463].

However, it is now recognized that this approach lacks clinical relevance, especially as it is based on a very dubious view of disease, and relies on the naturalistic paralogism [464] that confuses a judgment of fact with a normative judgment.

Finally, it appeals to a very limited view of evolution based exclusively on natural selection, and even more seriously, natural selection based exclusively on genes, a hypothesis that is now rejected [465].

The evolutionary metaphor identifies the body with a machine, and disease is then seen as a flaw in an otherwise perfect or near perfect mechanism.

The human body is badly, very badly designed. Why has natural selection left our bodies with traits that make us susceptible to disease? Why do people frequently get infections because of the suppression of the immune system? Why do our bodies lack the vitamin that accounts for millions of cases of scurvy, when cats can produce vitamin C but humans cannot? Life and the human body are far messier and more improvised than adaptationists would have us believe [466].

Moreover, natural selection is a tautology: it hardly seems explanatory to say that the reason various organisms have survived is that they were fittest if, by definition, the fittest are those that survive. On the one hand, it is assumed a priori that an organism's characteristics or traits are present because they enabled its ancestors to adapt better and were therefore selected because they were useful. On the other hand, any feature of a creature that attracts our attention must be useful or must have an adaptive advantage because it has been selected. This viciously circular reasoning implies that traits were selected because they were adapted, and conversely, that they are adapted because they were selected [467].

Voltaire's Dr Pangloss saw a purpose in everything: "*Everything is made for the best*". This Panglossian fallacy has led to a systematic application of natural selection to the problems of medicine, covering sex, menstruation, pregnancy, allergy, cancer, senescence, mental disorders, infectious diseases, etc. [468] Characteristics and traits must undoubtedly be given an adaptationist explanation, for everything that exists, exists because it is for the best: suffering, illness, vomiting, fever, coughing, diarrhea, or the claim that the male immune system is weakened by testosterone, all of which is supposed to serve to maximize the reproductive success of our genes.

This common misconception is pure speculation without any empirical support. It is assumed that the majority of pleasant or unpleasant physical or emotional characteristics serve some yet unidentified purpose, since Mother Nature, under the guise of natural selection, never proceeds in vain: "... *we have gained a better understanding of how the organism has been shaped by natural selection*," writes Randolph Nesse. The latter pushes the aporia to the point of defining disease not from clinical realities, but by deduction from his peremptory hypothetical system, and too bad if medicine is wrong! [469].

Of course, there is no problem with Darwinism and with its idea of natural selection operating on spontaneous variations as a mechanism explaining the journey from single-cell creatures to the human organism. However, the dogmatic hyperdadaptationist programme is a new religion, which was named Darwinitis by the physician and philosopher Raymond Tallis [470] and has often been denounced in the literature [471]. Darwin himself warned that "natural selection has been the principal, but not the exclusive, means of modification" [472]. Raymond Tallis complains of "the mistaken belief that Darwinism forces us to accept the Darwinite claim that everything about people is explained in terms of biological evolution" [473].

These medical explanations are governed by anthropological assumptions about Paleolithic man's past, so that we run the risk of idealizing the lives of our Stone Age ancestors, rather than appealing to real causes, as determined by current clinical or epidemiological investigations.

However, we now know that humans are still evolving. In natural selection, or "survival of the fittest", characteristics that improve survival are more likely to be passed on to the next generation.

It is not a disfigurement of Darwinism to reject this dogmatic, simplistic, and untestable scheme that attributes causal and explanatory sufficiency to natural selection alone and claims that all characteristics of organisms are either optimal characteristics or are specifically produced by the forks of ultra-Darwinian selection.

Why do these authors ignore "genetic drift", "sampling error" or migration to find a habitat in which an unchanged trait improves fitness, which may help explain adaptation? [474] Should we not consider a more pluralistic, Neo-Darwinist approach, including genetic drift or survival of the fittest, whereby a gene can become dominant in a population by pure chance; developmental biases; horizontal transmission of DNA; epigenetic inheritance that is more frequent than previously thought; and the separability of the current utility of a trait from the evolutionary reasons for the existence of that trait?

The famous Darwinian, Stephen Gould, and the geneticist and philosopher, Richard Lewontin [475], illustrate this misuse of natural selection as an explanatory tool by quoting Robert Wright, who argues that our penchant for sweetness was designed for an environment in which fruit existed, but sweets did not. Gould comments: "*This ranks with pure cocktail party speculation; Wright presents no neurological evidence for a brain module for sweetness, nor any paleontological data on ancestral feeding. This "just story" cannot therefore be considered a "classic example of adaptation" in a sense that deserves the name science.*"

Gould and Lewontin's paper "*The spandrel of San Marco and the Panglossian paradigm*" is a very influential paper which indicates how certain non-adaptive features inevitably result from the process of natural selection. The evolutionary process imposes a series of sequelae on any adaptive change.

These sequels—tympanums or spandrels in the terminology of the article (a term borrowed from architectural design for the pendentives of San Marco in Venice)—refer to a class of forms and spaces that appear as by-products of architectural constraint, not as an adaptation for direct utility in themselves. The design of the spandrels of St Mark's Basilica is "*so elaborate, harmonious and determined that we are tempted to regard it as the starting point of all analysis, as the cause in some sense of the surrounding architecture*". They then argue that this would be inappropriate, as the spandrels themselves were an architectural necessity that "*provided a space in which the mosaicists worked*".

"The organizations cannot optimize each part without imposing costs on the others. The notion of 'trade-offs' is introduced, and organisms are interpreted as the best compromises between competing demands."

Evolutionary biology needs such an explicit idea for features that appear as side-effects, rather than adaptations, regardless of their later *exapted* utility, namely a function that was not acquired by natural selection and for which it was not originally adapted. Darwin himself provides examples of highly useful functions that were not selected for, so there is evidence for a non-selectionist hypothesis [476].

Strict Darwinism often reduces the process of adaptation to all aspects of the evolution of a characteristic. The primary mechanism of natural selection is then seen as a direct causal basis for the whole sequence.

On the other hand, spandrels do not appear as mere by-products of architecture, but may regulate or dominate the late history of a lineage because of their ability to coapt to later utility.

Let us add that the constant recourse in philosophy of medicine to natural selection is a fallacious explanation. It is the genetic fallacy, the fallacy of confusing temporal or historical origin with logical nature [477].

Lewontin is concerned with the potentially misleading label of '*adaptation*'. Focusing on the parallels between natural selection and natural theology, one is tempted to think of selection as akin to a 'blind watchmaker', i.e., selection as a craftsman shaping organic form to meet environmental problems [478].

Explanatory adaptation is merely a statement of explanatory interest, an interest that we should not feel obliged to share, but which is sometimes better understood as a heuristic rather than an empirical hypothesis [479].

According to Schaffner, although medicine may use teleological discourse in its attempts to develop a mechanistic picture of human functioning, teleology is only heuristic and can be dispensed with altogether when the mechanistic explanation of a given organ or process is complete [480].

Incidentally, Wittgenstein also questioned uncertain historical explanations in anthropology [481]. While he respected the contribution of the new paradigm proposed by Darwin: "The real merit of a Copernicus or a Darwin was not the discovery of a true theory but that of a new and fruitful way of seeing" [482], he confided to his friend Drury in 1949 that he believed Darwin's theory to be correct. In 1949 he confided to his friend Drury that he believed Darwinian theory to be false. Wittgenstein's somewhat surprising attitude to evolution has complex sources that are clearly analyzed by Silvia di Cesare [483].

Chapter 10
The Origin and Foundation of Medicine

Omnis determonatio est negatio

Spinoza

Abstract This chapter covers the ontology of medicine. Medicine is not initially based on the concept of disease, but rather on actual or potential biological negativities, whether acute or chronic, such as physical or mental suffering, disrupting disabilities, severe signs or symptoms, or death. Normal and abnormal are contradictories, but normal and pathological are contraries.

Normality is multiple and is defined counterfactually. The pathological has logical priority over being normal.

Keywords Medical ontology · Normal · Abnormal · Pathological · Primacy of the pathological

Archê, according to Aristotle, is the first thing, the principle of what consists of something and of what follows from it. Origin (from the Latin *origo*, 'the source') is that which is first in the sense of that which is the source of a reality, process, or knowledge, the beginning or initial moment of the appearance of a thing.

Foundationalism is the epistemological theory that knowledge rests on a foundation of absolute certainty. Wittgenstein's conception of philosophy seemed to make it ill-suited to provide such a foundation for science. However, his last book, *On Certainty,* proposes a new kind of foundationalism, whereby our knowledge depends on a foundation of certainty. The foundation is that on which a knowledge or theory rests, that which is first in the logical order of things, and which is the reason for the existence of a phenomenon, its justification.

Wittgenstein writes: "*If the true is what is grounded, then the ground is not true or false." and "At the foundation of well-founded belief is unfounded belief*" [484].

Without shared attitudes towards medicine, with its theoretical and pragmatic dimensions, communication between human beings and health care would be impossible. It is important, for example, that almost everyone agrees almost all the time on what pain, disability or suffering are.

L. Karhausen, *The Fragility of Philosophy of Medicine*, Philosophy and Medicine 147, https://doi.org/10.1007/978-3-031-41633-0_10

What is the basis of medicine, not historically and culturally, but conceptually? What are the premises that support the logical architecture of medicine and give rise to medical science, medical practice, and public health? Thoreau asserted that "there is a solid ground everywhere" [485]. Where and how does the origin of medicine separate from biology?

10.1 Not Diseases

For most, if not all, books, texts, or treatises on the philosophy of medicine, the central concept of clinical medicine is disease. "Medical science, it seems, has disease as its object," writes Maël Lemoine [486]. Horacio Fabrega argues that "medicine, as an institution of society, is defined in terms of its interest in disease". Fred Gifford adds, "The concepts of health and disease seem to be quite fundamental to medicine, for we see medicine as having as its goals the diagnosis, prevention and cure of disease or the achievement of health" [493]. Jeremy R. Simon in a lengthy and detailed essay on medical ontology [487, 488], states that a primary desideratum in any field of philosophy is a clear understanding of the entities under consideration: "In the philosophy of medicine, this presupposes an understanding of the nature of individual illnesses. For Jacob Stegenga, disease is a fundamental issue in medicine" [489]. Corbellini, at the end of his book *History and Theory of Health and Disease*, writes an appendix on "the epistemological evolution of medicine" which essentially covers the concept of disease [490]. From Hippocrates and Galen until the second half of the twentieth century, the term—if not the concept—of 'disease' has been the essence of medicine. All in all, for most authors, health and disease are the primary point of view to be grasped.

However, is this idea relevant or is it premature?

In contrast, Peter Schwarz, professor of medicine at Indiana University, argues that diseases are not interesting or sufficiently coherent theoretical entities, and that there is no general underlying concept of disease in the biomedical sciences [491]. "*Doctors do not treat diseases, they treat patients,*" writes Eric Cassell [492]. People do not complain about diseases but about unexplained pain, suffering, anxiety, symptoms, or somatic signs, which are not necessarily manifestations of disease. Diseases are not at the heart of medicine any more than constellations are at the heart of astronomy.

Health is not the absence of disease, because disease is only a fraction, often a small fraction, of the conditions seen in clinical medicine. Several studies have shown that in 50–79% of all patients presenting to a family doctor, no evidence of a specific organic diagnosis could be found [493]. During the twentieth century, patients have become increasingly anxious about their health and more willing to consult their doctor. The so-called iceberg of symptoms instead of the iceberg of disease is becoming a major new socio-medical phenomenon [494].

What distinguishes medicine from biology? Unlike these two disciplines, the dividing line between them is not part of the furniture of the world.

Medicine, above all, needs a set of rules and criteria that separate normal from pathological characteristics. Concludes Eric Cassell: "Knowing the diseases, in the traditional sense, is not nearly as important as knowing the pathophysiology" [495].

Overall, these standards are medical conventions and are therefore neither true nor false, but rather correct or incorrect. Certainly, once adopted, the norms become part of clinical medicine and the grammar of medical language: the fact that they are then stored in medical texts and are constantly used in medical care reifies them and gives them a descriptive status, so that they become true or false.

In short, what distinguishes biology from medicine is that the former is descriptive, and the latter both descriptive and normative.

Medical thinking is based on the sequence of two tacit conventions, of opposite bases, which create the possibility of medical care.

First, it divides biological features into good and bad clinical manifestations, between harm, injury, suffering, and their absence; consequently, it decides what is normal and what is pathological and presents the medical topography along an asymmetrical spectrum in which pathological features have a logical factual priority. The brute fact of suffering, disability and harmful, or potentially harmful, biological conditions directly affecting the body or mind is legitimately admitted at the outset: it is the gateway to medicine. These conditions are bad or aversive, have serious consequences for the patient and call for help [496].

Then, a second convention reverses the order of priority: the norms of normality called health, physiology or anatomy and the need to maintain or restore normality then have epistemic and pragmatic priority over abnormal and pathological features.

Having recognized the existence of suffering, infirmity, complaints and handicaps, clinical medicine was born with the decision to divide biological characteristics into normal and pathological. Maël Lemoine writes that: "... is not the detrimental character of a condition really the only criterion of the pathological?" [497]. If the demarcation that separates the normal from the pathological is medical and not sociological (how could it be?), normal and pathological characteristics, once described, become factual, but the dividing line between them is not: it is a tacit agreement, so that the attribution of these two terms is conventional, normative and prescriptive, and therefore neither true nor false; this convention is anchored by the inherently negative and value-laden effects: the abnormal characteristics are the core of the prior reference and the normal characteristics represent the contrast reference.

From this grammatical perspective, these bivalent medical norms, and the boundary between them, although based on descriptions, are not part of the basic inventory of the real world but are prudential and deontic. Normative provisions are derived from the consensus generated by medical practice, so that more or fewer universal rules are established, and maintained by collectively controlling and sanctioning their individual tendencies. Consensus makes norms objective, i.e., it is an external and impersonal source of constraint for the individual.

This demarcation is so specific to medicine that it could be considered as one of its criteria: medicine, the human activity, is concerned with identifying the pathological by separating it from the counterfactual normal. Thus, if we were to remove or deduce from biological reality every abnormal feature or pathological process, there would remain a remainder, namely a default position called 'normality', usually called 'health'. At this stage, physiology, anatomy, or biochemistry would be true by default and based on the absence of pathological features. This is the starting point of the bottom-up ontology of medicine, what Broadbent calls the metaphysical position [498].

Ultimately, the first ontological position is to introduce and impose, for prudential reasons, the 'empirical and natural'—albeit false—descriptions of the biological world into conventional medical norms by dividing the biological domain into normal and pathological. Although this first position is among biological processes, its conventional division may be correct or incorrect but has no objective residence in the biological world. Therefore, abnormality is fundamental, and normality is defined negatively as contradictory to abnormality.

10.2 Are Symptoms in Medicine Private Objects?

Pain, Wittgenstein observes, is a feeling. Since it is a feeling, we do not generally test it. We do not challenge someone when they say they are in pain.

Not only do we not usually challenge statements of pain, but a fortiori we do not challenge the person making the statement, whereas we may, for example, challenge an obese patient when he or she says he or she is eating very little.

We cede to others the authority to determine if, and when, and to what extent, they suffer. If we challenge them, we question their sincerity. Pain, like most symptoms, is associated with incorrigibility. Wittgenstein reminds us that, given the meaning of the word 'pain' in our language, expressions such as 'I don't know if I am in pain' are meaningless.

Pain is an example of a sensation or symptom that we are tempted to regard as an inner object whose name is the word 'pain'. But Wittgenstein points out that pain and other sensations are not such objects, nor are they neurological objects. The grammatical facts do not require any explanation.

According to Wittgenstein, one does not use words such as 'pain', 'headache', 'thirst', fatigue, and so on, in the same way as one uses words to designate objects. It is therefore a mistake to think of symptoms as objects of a particular type, or of an ordinary physical type, which have a size, weight, shape, place, and so on. They do not refer to objects in the ordinary sense at all, not even to imaginary objects.

You can mistake a fox for a dog. But when you are in pain, there is no process for discovering that you are in pain. Nor can one mistake the sensation of pain, although it is sometimes difficult to characterize a sensation one experiences, one cannot fail to feel pain, but one cannot fail to see a bird flying past my window.

Wittgenstein [499] asks whether we can imagine a language whose individual words *"refer to what can only be known to the speaker, to his immediate private sensations. Another person cannot therefore understand this language"*. He argues that we cannot imagine such a 'private language' that would be exclusively about my symptoms. The implication of *the private language argument* is that there can be no language invented by and intelligible to a single individual. This follows from Wittgenstein's view that language is essentially public.

This raises many questions, starting with "How do words refer to feelings?", to which part of Wittgenstein's answer is that verbal expression of pain replaces and does not describe [500] crying, so that language is not "private" [501].

Pain is an example of a sensation that could be considered an inner object with the word "pain" as its name. He maintains that pain and other sensations are not such objects. He denies that pain is 'a nothing', but he also denies that it is something. Wittgenstein's argument refutes the very possibility of a language that is in principle incomprehensible to everyone except the person whose language it is: it would be a private language that describes his or her inner experiences, and whose vocabulary would be defined by sensations to which only that person has access. There can be no language consisting of such words for inner objects of experience, and no language can include such words. The words of a private language, which would be the boxed contents of each speaker's head, would have no real meaning.

It is a false assumption that one must learn about pain, anxiety, or fear "from one's own case", and that the thing to observe is not one's behaviour, but rather something "inside": this would mean that one notes something in oneself that one calls "pain", "anxiety" or "fear", and then tries to deduce from it the presence of the same thing in others [502]. There is no process for finding out that I have pain or itch.

Wittgenstein does not deny that if someone suffers pain, "they feel the same as I have often felt." What he does deny is the implication that this reference to "the same thing" explains something; it explains what it means to attribute pain to another person according to the argument of analogy; the meaning of "He is in pain" is given by assuming that he has the same feeling as I have when I am in pain. The meaning of the word 'pain' for me establishes and serves as a reference. But if Wittgenstein is right, this is not a meaning at all.

Wittgenstein rejects the idea that pain is the name of a certain kind of sensation by an act of inner ostension and a pointing object. Since the word 'pain' is not related to the type of sensation involved in the ostension, it denotes nothing at all; 'pain' is not a label.

How, then, is it related to the sensations we have used to speak?

There is an asymmetry between the 1st person and 3rd person concepts which has important consequences. It seems that we know our own experiences, while we must infer those of others. To say "I know I am in pain" is a logical and meaningful proposition, but it does not make sense because I do not know it and do not know it. It is not knowledge. Knowledge is related to doubt and certainty, learning and discovery, motives, and confirmation. These notions cannot be applied to my own pain.

Wittgenstein argues that the proper way to deal with the question of how a word names or refers is to describe its acquisition and use. If the remark "You learned the concept of 'pain' when you learned language" [503] is taken as a key remark, then the central point of the private language argument is that there can be no meaning without the possibility of telling whether a word's use is correct or not, and that this possibility cannot exist outside of a public—not private—use of words, a regular practice against which one can tell whether a word is being used correctly or not.

Wittgenstein suggests that first-person statements should be seen as like natural non-verbal and behavioural expressions of psychological states. For example, "My leg hurts" should be equated with crying, limping, holding one's leg. By uttering the sentence, one can make a statement: it has a contradiction; it is true or false; by uttering it, one is lying or telling the truth; and so on.

This approach has two important merits. First, it breaks the hold on us of the question "How does one know when to say, 'My leg hurts'?", for in the light of the analogy, this question will be as absurd as the question "How does one know when to cry, limp or hold one's leg?"

Secondly, it explains how the utterance of a psychological sentence in the first person by another person can matter to us, even though it is not an identification—for in the light of the analogy, it will matter as much as the natural behaviour that serves as our preverbal criterion of the psychological states of others. Wittgenstein says that "one possibility" is that talking about pain is a substitute for the moaning and grimacing that is the natural expression of pain [504].

Wittgenstein's view provides an answer to this problem. The rules for the use of 'pain', he says, are public rules, which apply in the same way when speaking of myself or others; there are not two sets of rules for such expressions, one governing self-registration and the other governing registration with the other of the states in question. Therefore, the reasons why I can say that someone else is in pain are provided by their behaviour and by my understanding of the rules for using the word 'pain'.

10.3 The Trajectory from Suffering to Disease

Pathos is defined by Aristotle [505]: "*The painful and destructive evils are death in its various forms, bodily injuries and afflictions, old age, diseases, famine*". "Suffering, which we can define as an action that involves destruction or pain, e.g., death," seems to play a role in the structure of empirical medical knowledge like that of axioms in deductive reasoning.

Wittgenstein writes: "*I imagine, then, that everyone says of himself that he knows what pain is only from his own,*" *and he adds:* "*To represent the pain of others on the model of one's own is not so easy, for I have to represent pains that I do not feel from pains that I do feel*" [506].

Firstly, suffering is the starting point of medicine since we know it directly and not through anything else [507].

Secondly, suffering is an intrinsic biological evil, whether physical or mental; it is unpleasant, disruptive, and worthless. Identifying which of the abnormal biological characteristics are harmful, or potentially harmful, i.e., which are termed 'pathological', is the fundamental convention of medical thinking. Ellen K. Feder argues: "*At the centre of medical knowledge is the distinction between 'normal' and 'abnormal'*" [508].

Third, the occurrences of suffering and intrinsic biological negativities are linked to the need for interventions. The obligation to deal with suffering, "writes Eric Cassell,"goes back to antiquity [509]. Aristotle argued that the main aspect of prudence, or practical wisdom (phronesis), lies not in the realm of knowledge but rather in that of action.

Reznek [510] was the first, but also the only one for whom a person P has a pathological condition C, if and only if C is an abnormal condition that requires medical intervention, and which, under normal circumstances, makes P less able to live a good or worthwhile life.

And this is how medicine begins.

10.4 Normal or Abnormal

It has often been observed that the logical symmetry of negative and affirmative propositions in logic masks a fundamental asymmetry in natural language. It was Plato who first observed in The Sophist that negative sentences are less specific and informative and have less value than affirmative sentences. The ontological, epistemological, psychological, and grammatical priority of affirmatives over negatives is supported by Aristotle: 'The affirmative proposition is prior to the negative and better known than the negative (since the affirmation explains the denial just as the fact of being is prior to the fact of not being)" [511]. And for Thomas Aquinas: "The affirmative utterance is prior to the negative for three reasons... As regards vocal sound, the affirmative utterance is prior to the negative because it is simpler, because the negative utterance adds a negative particle to the affirmative. About thought, the affirmative enunciation, which means composition by the intellect, is prior to the negative, which means division... As regards the thing, the affirmative enunciation, which signifies being, is prior to the negative, which signifies not being, for the having of something is naturally prior to its deprivation" [512].

Philosophers of medicine locate this semantic asymmetry as the assertion that every negation presupposes a corresponding affirmative, but not vice versa. This position leads to the "paradox of the negative judgment": if a positive statement refers to or corresponds to a positive fact, to what state of affairs does a negative statement refer or correspond?

Negation has also been analyzed in various ways as a modality, a propositional attitude, and a speech act. The danger here is to put the cart before the horse. For example, not all negation is speaker denial: in making this point, Godfried Frege emphasized embedded negation as in 'If not, then', and not all speaker denial is linguistic negation either. Given the repeated attempts over the centuries to liquidate or tame it—negation as positive difference, as dissimilarity or incompatibility, as falsity, as an admission of epistemic impoverishment, as an act of speech denial,—and its resistance to these attacks—negation is called the Rasputin of propositional calculation.

But the prototypical use of negation is indeed as a negation of a proposition attributable to, or at least considered by, someone reasonable in the context of discourse. Whereas the assertion usually introduces a proposition into the main discourse model [513], the negation—in its "primary use," its "most common use" according to Ayer [514], its "standard and primary use" according to Strawson [515]—is aimed at a proposition that is already in the discourse model or that can be considered by it.

If, however, we were to propose a rule here, it would contain the phrase "under normal circumstances". And we recognize normal circumstances, but we cannot describe them precisely. At most, we can describe a series of abnormal circumstances [516].

Wittgenstein observes: "*Can image and application therefore conflict? They can, insofar as the image leads us to expect a different use, because in general one makes such and such an application of this image.*"

"*I mean, here there is a normal case and an abnormal case.*"

"*The use of words is clearly prescribed to us only in normal cases. We know what we have to say in such and such a case, we have no doubt about it. But the more the case deviates from the normal, the more dubious that we have to say becomes. And if things were quite different from what they really are—if, for example, there were no characteristic expressions of pain, fear, joy, if the rule became the exception and the exception the rule, or if they both became phenomena of roughly the same frequency—our normal language games would lose their interest*" [517].

What for Boorse best defines medical normality is that functions have a range of normal values. He concludes, on the one hand, that what is normal corresponds to the functional design that is empirically typical of the species in question, i.e., is physiological [518].

On the other hand, what is pathological is identified with a sub-optimal functioning of the organism in relation to the functional design typical of its species.

There are major objections to these two statements.

The first is that *physiology is false* because it is a theoretical construct which is not empirical, and which assumes normality, i.e., appealing to physiology is circular: the language of physiology is supposed to be that of normality, so that what is physiological is normal.

The second is that most diseases and pathological processes are not sub-functions but abnormal functioning, such as cancers, autoimmune diseases like myasthenia gravis, multiple sclerosis or rheumatoid arthritis, and many mental disorders like schizophrenia.

What is normal is neither statistical nor empirical, as Boorse would have it, but grammatical. The different and multiple approaches that seek to define normality show that it is not an empirical notion and that it is impossible to propose a naturalistic definition of normality.

Physiologically normal systolic blood pressure—i.e., without any cardiovascular complications—is below 90 mm Hg, which is the threshold above which cardiovascular risk increases linearly [519]. A person with a systolic blood pressure of 90 mm

Hg would probably experience discomfort, dizziness, or fatigue, so that this physiologically normal blood pressure would be clinically unacceptable.

Antihypertensive treatment is beneficial even when blood pressure is normal [520].

Furthermore, a normal blood pressure may be normal either for the heart or for the brain. The normal blood pressure depends on which outcome we are most interested in since there is no one size fit. The investigations show that for a patient with a particular risk of stroke, more aggressive blood pressure lowering may be warranted than a patient with a particular risk for myocardial infarction. Identifying patients more at risk of one type of cardiovascular even than another can be very challenging [521].

The above highlights the vanity of basing medical concepts, and those of disease, on such an elusive and inherently contradictory notion as normality [522].

Canguilhem stated that the identification of the normal and the pathological presupposes an objective definition of the normal: without an objective definition of the normal, there is no starting point for the quantitative extension of the normal to the pathological. His mistake was to reverse the order of things: the identification of the normal and the pathological presupposes a definition of the pathological [523].

10.5 Distinguishing the Abnormal from the Pathological

"Normal and pathological were usually considered as opposites, but the notion of disease risk seems to introduce a continuity," writes Elodie Giroux.

However, in terms of logic, *normal and pathological are contradictories, while normal and abnormal are contraries*. This distinction, which the philosophy of medicine literature seems to ignore, allows us to distinguish the dichotomy of normal/pathological and the continuum of normal/abnormal. This distinction is well known in medicine, since the very essence of medical activity is to distinguish and decide what is pathological, i.e., what requires intervention, in the continuum of the abnormal. It may happen, as in the case of hypertension, that pathological levels of risk are chosen, but never, of course, continuity. Moreover, unlike diseases, medical standards are generally fairly constant throughout human history.

However, in the second half of the last century, medicine gradually became interested in quantitative or naturally continuous variables. However, medicine, driven by the need to intervene, needs single cut-off points; to remove vagueness and at the risk of being too rigid, it resorts to stipulative definitions or the decision to divide the range of abnormal traits into two (or more) pathological categories, each with a range of variability [524]. This conventional fiat, which is always subject to revision, classifies individuals into sick and not sick, those who need care and those who do not, those who are pathological and those who are normal. In this way, continuous and natural distributions are transformed into discrete categories.

To say that an abnormal state or process is pathological implies that it is intrinsically harmful. Being pathological is undesirable: it causes pain or unpleasant experiences and limits freedom of action, development, and growth.

In saying this, amusia is abnormal but never pathological, whereas anhedonia is abnormal and can become pathological.

This perhaps deserves a digression. Opposite terms can be *contraries* (like white and not white) if both cannot be true though they might both be false, so that one must be true and the other false: they have an opposite truth value. Hence, 'normal' is contradictory to 'abnormal': what is abnormal is not normal. In the case of two opposite terms (such as being white and one of the ways of being non-white, e.g., red), at least one of them is false and both cannot be true, but both can be false.

The terms normal and pathological are *contradictory*: they cannot both be true, but some features can be abnormal without being pathological, for example in the case of minor dermatological disorders such as lipomas, skin spots or angiomas. In this case, normal and pathological are opposites.

What is pathological is abnormal, but what is abnormal is not necessarily pathological. It is true, however, that the terms 'abnormal' and 'pathological' are often used as synonyms in medical language.

Being abnormal is progressive, while being pathological is dichotomous. Claude Bernard showed that abnormality may not be a discrete term but a scalar one, in which case there is a continuum of severity from healthy to very serious states. "Hence the importance," writes Wittgenstein, "of finding intermediate links" [525].

A kidney cyst is abnormal, but not pathological. Ventricular ectopic beats are abnormal: they always represent a premature depolarization of the ventricles, an abnormal electro-physiological process; although present in more than half of apparently normal people, they may be pathological, that is, evidence of a serious disturbance of the cardiac rhythm.

Abnormal is often regarded as a statistical concept, whereas pathology is a medical convention. Only statistical abnormalities that have adverse consequences are likely to be pathological. Abnormal is an open-textured, interval-valued predicate that admits degrees: it represents a continuum of negative, predictive, increasing consequences and a domain of medical uncertainty. If being abnormal is scalar, being pathological is non-scalar and stipulative. This distinction is essential because it allows us to separate a quantifiable phenomenon from a predicate which, unlike being abnormal, has a deontic status: it calls for a remedial intervention.

To call a biological or abnormal condition or process pathological implies that it is inherently harmful. To describe an unfavourable anatomical or functional characteristic as pathological means that it is detrimental to the interests of the well-being of the individual concerned, i.e., to his or her body or health in relation to what the condition would have been had the characteristic been absent. Pathological characteristics are tendencies or dispositions to deteriorate or decay; they are potential causes or pathways to disease. The claim that certain characteristics or processes are pathological is a modal claim, meaning that they are statistically harmful [526].

Confusing abnormal with pathological is a frequent source of unnecessary diagnoses and erroneous treatments.

It should be remembered that while pathological and non-pathological features are natural phenomena, the line between what is pathological and what is not is not in the inventory of the natural world. The result is that the meaning of the term 'pathological' is not a matter of nature but of convention.

Wittgenstein wrote: "*Good and evil enter the world only through the subject. And the subject is not a part of the world, but a limit of the world*" [527].

In short, pathological features are not identifiable in the biological world as pathological, but they are in our theoretical medical doctrines and medical grammar. They betray the distorting lenses through which medicine examines biological facts. But being pathological comes into play, so to speak, in an intentional context, because it is a mere convention, not a fact.

10.6 Normality Is Not a Biological But a Medical Concept

Normality is multiple. It is impossible to give a naturalistic definition of what is normal. The logical priority is what is abnormal or pathological because that is what defines the contours of what is normal.

For example, what is normal blood pressure?

Blood pressure may need to be modified according to the cardiovascular outcome for which the patient is most at risk. For a patient at particular risk of stroke, a more aggressive reduction may be warranted than a patient at particular risk of myocardial infarction.

A systolic/diastolic pressure of 140–155/70–80 mm Hg was associated with the lowest risk of all-cause mortality, compared with 110–120/85–90 mm Hg for myocardial infarction and 125–135/70–75 mm Hg for heart failure. In contrast, the association of systolic and diastolic blood pressure with stroke is linear, with lower values of both measures consistently associated with a lower risk of stroke.

It is probably inappropriate to adopt a single approach to blood pressure targets. The normal blood pressure target may depend on the outcome of interest: heart attack, heart failure or stroke. The aggressiveness with which we want to lower blood pressure could be influenced by whether a patient is at greater risk of a future stroke or cardiac event. The idea that one size fits all, but for blood pressure targets it is not appropriate [528]. There is no biological standard for blood pressure.

10.7 The Logical Priority of the Pathological

Medicine is based on a medical convention, the conventional distinction between the notions of normal and pathological, whereas being normal is the default position.

Being abnormal has the primary meaning because it has a certain logical priority over being normal. But it also has a psychological priority. Plato wrote: "Well, you must have heard people say, when they are ill, that nothing is more pleasant than to be well, though they never knew it before they were ill" [529].

Lars Bergström has proposed a principle of non-additivity of utility, which applies at the clinical level when physiological norms of normality prevail: a normally functioning heart does not compensate for a failing kidney. Biological negativities are additive: a patient with both heart disease and kidney failure is more severely affected than a patient developing only one disease. In contrast and in place of negative norms, positive norms, i.e., normal characteristics, are not additive: the principle of non-additivity of utility means that a normally functioning heart does not compensate for kidney failure.

This asymmetry between the normal and the abnormal underlines the priority of the pathological over the normal, i.e., they are not symmetrical in the additivity of their features.

Elisha Bartlett (1804–1835) added: "Pathology is not based on physiology... Our knowledge of the disease processes and susceptibilities of the various organs and tissues of the body cannot be deduced from our knowledge of their healthy processes.

Magna est vis instantiae negativae.

Contrary to popular opinion [530], norms in medical logic are negative. Several pairs of words, which are the cornerstone of medical systems, such as "normal" and "abnormal", "rational" and "irrational", "sick" and "cured", "anxiety" and "relief", "health" and "disease" or "life" and "death", show a significant asymmetry [531]. "*We feel pain, not the absence of pain*", writes Schopenhauer. The negative members of the above pairs are irreducible as well as more determinate, explicit and fundamental than the positive members, which are ill-defined and indicate derivative, secondary paths in the theoretical articulation of medical concepts. The factors and processes that make people suffer or disabled are better known and much more firmly rooted and classified than those that make them healthy. Death is a definable fact and there are lists of causes of death, but we rarely ask what the reasons for being alive are. Having something wrong: pain, disability or death are basic concepts that clarify the logic of the concept of 'pathological' [532]. And J.L. Austin suggests that "so often the abnormal illuminates the normal" [533].

In health and disease, pathology has the first word since it is conceptually prior to physiology. A normally functioning heart is not described as normal because of some benefit it provides, but simply because it does not cause harm; defining a certain function as normal implies the deprivation or absence of some painful or harmful characteristics that result from it. The oldest Greek biology books presented "the evolution of physiology and pathology and they tended to start with the sick man (with pathology) and from there learned the normal constitution of men" [534].

On this point, physiology at this stage is true by default and is based on the absence of abnormalities or diseases. In medical parlance, physiology is true *ceteris paribus*, by deliberate omission, so that it is in fact false: it describes non-existent processes to which real processes can be compared, classified, and aligned in terms of similarity. Physiology echoes Newton's seventeenth century ideals of natural order, such as his principle of inertia, i.e., his first law of motion, which was an abstract paradigm of natural motion, never encountered in the real world.

It provides us, "writes Toulmin," [535] rather with a criterion by which to tell in what respect the motion of an organ calls for an explanation... Only if a body were left completely to itself would it move regularly along a straight line, and no real body is ever placed in this extreme position. And this concept of the 'natural course of events' is given in negative terms: positive complications produce positive effects and are invoked to explain deviations from the natural ideal, rather than conformity to it. That said, the appearance of words like 'inert' and 'inertia' in our theories is perhaps significant. For they are essentially negative terms, indicating how things will behave on their own if nothing is done to them from outside. If left to their own devices, things will follow their "natural" course."

Medicine does not maintain that one must be normal: what is desirable is not the condition of carrying normal traits but rather the condition of not having pathological traits. This implies, it seems to me, that normality is privative, i.e., it is constructed counterfactually because it corresponds to the absence of abnormal characteristics. On the contrary, to be harmful or prejudicial means to affect someone's health unfavourably, which is not the same thing as not affecting it favourably: this is what is logically primitive.

To put it bluntly, medicine is primarily concerned with suffering and the bodily or mental states that may result from thwarting prudential needs. The relief of suffering makes a stronger claim than the promotion of positive outcomes such as happiness or health. Public health itself has been governed much more by threat avoidance than by goal seeking [536].

10.8 Medicine as a System and the Pathological Is Its Foundation

Wittgenstein repeatedly emphasizes the diversity of human practices and fields of discourse. On several occasions he gives examples of different systems. He uses the term 'system' as a system of proof and verification [537]; methods of confirmation and investigation that are applicable in one domain are not applicable in another [538]. If we are to accept a picture of knowledge as composed of different belief systems, in the sense that geography, history, biology, medicine or the social sciences, for example, form different systems of proof and verification whose rules depend on the kind of thing being studied in each case, then these systems cannot be seen as discrete and discontinuous: facts established in, say, the history of biology can influence what is believed in medicine.

In scientific investigation, there are strict rules and propositions indicating which discoverable facts can be transformed into standards of description. As such, they play a constitutive role in the method of our investigation. All tests and confirmations take place within a system [539]. And this system is not based on what we can know to be true, but on activities and practices. Moreover, the truth of certain empirical propositions belongs to our frame of reference. If the meaning of a proposition is to be given in terms of verification, then, unless we are going to be led into an infinite regress of verifying conditions, there must be some point at which the process comes to an end. There is reason for supposing, then, that both knowledge and meaning must be grounded by reference to some set of basic propositions, propositions which are in some way self-validating. At the base of every well-formulated belief, Wittgenstein showed us, is a belief that is unfounded: "... in the river the bed of thoughts can move...", but "the riverbank is partly made of hard rock, susceptible to no or imperceptible alteration..." [540].

For our normal propositions, concerning the formation of an image or a mode of action, to work, other propositions must be solid. They function as hinges on which other propositions turn [541]. Thus, the pathological and the biological negativities, which contain the rules on which medicine is based, can be compared to hinges [542].

10.9 The Case of Hypertension

Since the distribution of blood pressure in the population is continuous, an arbitrary cut-off point is needed to define hypertension [543]. A person with a systolic blood pressure of 160 mm Hg is considered hypertensive and a person with a systolic blood pressure of 110 mm Hg is considered normotensive; but in between these two extremes there are penumbral cases in which it is not possible to say whether the blood pressure is normal or not.

Since the likelihood of cardiovascular complications is exponentially related to the increase in blood pressure over the entire range and without a threshold, it is important to define the level above which intervention is required [544].

There are people at high cardiovascular risk but with normal or slightly elevated blood pressure. Conversely, there are people with blood pressure above the current treatment threshold who have an overall low risk of cardiovascular disease.

This shows how physiological norms, although conventional and yet remaining so, can change under the pressure of new evidence. If the guidelines had lowered the systolic to 110 mm Hg, very few people with suspected hypertension would be missed, but many normal individuals would be misclassified as hypertensive; conversely, if the systolic pressure limit was set at 140 mm Hg, a smaller proportion of suspected hypertensives would be misclassified as normal, but a larger fraction of normals would be classified as hypertensive.

Thus, translating quantitative variables into qualitative variables by establishing a cut-offline involves trade-offs: to avoid misclassifying normal individuals, one must accept not including all abnormal individuals; conversely, to be sure of identifying all abnormal individuals, one must accept misclassifying as abnormal and increasing the fraction of normal individuals. The choice of the best cut-off value for hypertension becomes quite delicate when the distributions of the normal and pathological population overlap.

In short, in the case of a discrete variable, we usually know whether it is pathological; but if it is not, we consider a wide range of clinical, epidemiological, and statistical information, then assess what risks correspond to the different levels of a continuous variable, and finally decide what our operational threshold of pathology, i.e., intervention, will be: this is how a disease is defined.

Imprecision is inherent in qualitative predicates; they are scalar adjectives and correspond to a range of properties that occur in degrees; they involve comparative properties such as certain clinical manifestations (height, blood pressure), as well as most characteristics identified by diagnostic procedures, including signs and symptoms (e.g., BUN level, length of P-Q segments in ECG), functional abilities and most behavioural characteristics. In addition, some pathological features such as cataract, diabetes mellitus or depressive manifestations are also scalar concepts. We can generally classify them by comparing them to a conventional standard of normality.

- From this perspective, hypertension does not come in ontological blocks: there are infinitely different and graded levels of hypertension, with a corresponding continuum of potential harm. The new AHA guidelines and the 2017 American Heart Association Scientific Sessions recommend new treatment goals [545]:
  - Normal: Systolic blood pressure below 120 mm Hg, and diastolic blood pressure below 80 mm Hg.
  - High: Systolic between 120 and 129 and diastolic below 80.
  - Stage 1 hypertension: mean systolic blood pressure of 130–139 mm Hg, and diastolic blood pressure of 80–89 mm Hg (previously called prehypertension).
  - Stage 2 hypertension: mean systolic blood pressure of 140 mm Hg or more and diastolic blood pressure of 90 mm Hg or more.
  - Elderly patients: Elderly patients have the same treatment target as younger adults, although several health authorities (American College of Physicians and Academy of Family Physicians) have recommended a target systolic blood pressure of less than 150 mm Hg for the elderly; it should be 100 plus the patient's age.

10.10 The Case of Obesity

Obesity is, apart from a few exceptions, considered as a risk prankster and not as a disease. It is considered medically and sociologically abnormal [546].

However, a recent study by Anika Zembic of the Institute of Human Nutrition in Potsdam-Rehbruecke, has identified obese individuals, without diabetes or hypertension, who have no increased risk of cardiovascular disease. This is metabolically healthy obesity. Based on this new definition, 42% of participants in the third National Health and Nutrition Survey and 19% of participants in the UK Biobank survey do not have an increased risk of cardiovascular mortality compared to individuals with a normal, healthy body weight.

This means that individuals with metabolically healthy obesity may progress over time to unhealthy obesity through weight gain, ageing or lack of exercise.

10.11 Harmful and Pathological

Harm, whether caused or suffered by an organism, is a defining or essential characteristic of pathological character. It is logically impossible for a biological "harm" or "harmful act" to apply to a characteristic to which the term "pathological" does not apply. And it is also logically impossible for the term "pathological" to apply to a characteristic to which the term "harm" would not apply. The term "pathological" refers to a deleterious biological manifestation or state, namely a harmful state.

However, being harmful differs from being pathological in that a harmful condition, process, or situation is itself harmful, whereas being pathological is not pathological. A harmful thing, such as a disease, is aversive for two reasons: it produces harm and it is itself a bad condition, namely the condition of a person who has suffered harm, insofar as it results from causes that are harmful.

However, 'harm' is a term in common use, while 'pathological' is a theoretical term; the former refers to a process or the outcome of a process, the latter to a norm. Damage is gradual but being pathological is bivalent. The term 'pathological' is opposed to 'normal', but harm is opposed to 'well-being', 'benefit' or 'need satisfaction'. The notion of harm seems more conceptually fundamental than that of pathological, in that it is independent of our representations. Being pathological attributes a convention, whereas being harmful, so to speak, is an observation.

A consequence follows from this analysis. The pathological character is attributed in the presence of an aggregate or emergent sum of disparate harmful processes or situations or states of affairs. "Our 'empirical propositions' do not form a homogeneous mass," writes Wittgenstein" [547].

10.12 Biological Negativities Are Normative

Empirical propositions are descriptive since they describe states of affairs, but normative propositions are not descriptive but are necessary because they express grammatical rules. They are neither true nor false, but correct or incorrect. They express the reasons why we act and can only be justified within the framework of the medical clinic in general, which sets its own standards.

Abnormal and pathological are terms of family resemblance insofar as they are assigned in clinical medicine because of overlapping similarities.

Abnormal or pathological represent negative values, based on suffering or incapacity, and they are transcendental, as they cannot be in the world, but are located outside it [548, 549]. Values, Wittgenstein said, "cannot be found in the world", which itself is neither good nor bad [550]. They are grammatically constructed and publicly discernible. They are part of a medical activity, a form of life.

Medicine was born out of a need to alleviate or prevent physical or mental suffering, and in the course of its history it has extended the concept of suffering to interpersonal relationships.

What we call David Hume's guillotine is that *one can never derive an ought from an is*. One can never derive from purely biological or physiological data what is abnormal or pathological. The distinction between normal and abnormal, between normal and pathological, is therefore not a scientific one. This distinction is the very foundation of medicine. And these foundations are not descriptive, but are the expression of conventions and attitudes, even if medical language is inevitably bastardised since the practice of the clinic makes it both descriptive and normative.

That value judgements and factual judgements may be indistinguishable in terms of evidence and defensibility is entirely consistent with the distinction between value predicates and factual predicates. Whenever value norms are introduced and the judgment is about them, we have value judgments and not only factual judgments.

If evaluative and non-evaluative predicates are distinguished according to their role in our conceptual theories—in particular, according to whether their use involves the use of normative considerations—then it is quite possible to argue that evaluative predicates are equivalent in extension to sets of purely descriptive predicates (i.e., non-evaluative predicates) and while they are nonetheless distinguishable from these purely descriptive predicates. This means that it is not necessary, in providing for the distinction of value judgements, to admit a separate use of these judgements, as emotivists and imperativists demand; this distinction is sufficiently supported by the conceptual difference between the two kinds of predicates.

The common territory shared by the overlapping normal and pathological distributions represents the fringe, a twilight zone of dubious application, which includes borderline cases, an intermediate level known as "pre-hypertensive", the domain of the abnormal. Similarly, several other measures, such as glucose tolerance and diabetes, or intraocular pressure and glaucoma, or osteopenia and osteoporosis, can be related to the number of cases in which the disease in question is present or absent, resulting in two partially overlapping probability curves.

Thus, translating quantitative variations into qualitative variations by drawing a line of demarcation involves compromises: to avoid misclassifying normal individuals, one must accept not to include all abnormal individuals; conversely, to ensure that all abnormal individuals are identified, one must accept to misclassify them as abnormal and increase the fraction of normals.

Henrik Von Wright points out that "the relationship between the functioning organ and its effects on the body is a causal and therefore extrinsic relationship. But the relationship between the poor quality of the effects and the poor quality of the organ whose functioning is responsible for those effects is a logical and therefore intrinsic relationship [551]. If this is the case, then what makes a dysfunction pathological is grammatical in nature and constitutes what we mean by dysfunction.

When a cardiologist, because of signs of dyspnea and peripheral oedema, diagnoses a case of heart failure, this relationship between the dysfunction, as a cardiac disorder, and its negative consequences, signs, and symptoms, is not causal, but grammatical: it is constitutive of the clinical disorder insofar as it has to do with the meanings of the terms "abnormal", "pathological", "disorder", "dysfunction" and the like. The relationship between a failing organ and its effects is thus both causal, i.e., extrinsic, and grammatical; but the relationship between an unpleasant sensation of dyspnea and cardiac decompensation is intrinsic. This again reflects the primacy of negativities in the structure of medical representations.

Medical treatises often end with a very long list of normal laboratory values ranging from acetocholinesterase levels in the blood to vitamin levels in the serum. These figures are what Wittgenstein calls rules. These rules do not answer the "Why?" question of the natural or medical sciences, but rather questions like "Why do it?" or "Why can I?" or "Why must we?"

The word "rules" brings something to games, legal or medical practices. The most obvious way to appeal to a rule is to refer to it explicitly: "This is against the rules". Another characteristic of rules is their generality. Finally, rules are governed by rules of meaning: a rule gives us reasons to behave in a certain way [552–554].

Chapter 11
Functions, Malfunctions, and Teleology

> *Physiology extends its very limited empirical knowledge of the purposes of the members of an organic body by a principle inspired by pure reason alone.*
>
> Kant

Abstract Machines are intentional devices. Yet, functions usually explained teleologically, even though the consequence of a trait cannot explain why that trait is present. Kant admitted that this interpretation is a project in nature of our desires and John Searle indicated that the concept of function is always relative to an observer. A distinction should be mad between functional role and functional capacity. Diseases are one thing malfunction is another.

Keywords Functions · Malfunctions · Teleology · Functional role · functional capacity

The term "function" comes from "fung": to do. It is the role of an organ, a part of an organ, a physiological activity, or a mental module in an organism. The best definition of function in medicine would be a list of functions described in physiological texts. However, the function of a constituent part or process in an organism consists in the role it plays or is intended to play, and in its contribution to the overall body economy: the function of the pancreas is explained by saying what it does for the organism.

Contrast this with Boorse, who in his naturalistic approach defines function as the causal contribution of something to a goal in a teleological system. According to Boorse, functions contribute to needs, goals and objectives [555]. This naturalistic theory of function in biology and statistical normality is perfectly compatible when applied to machines, suggesting that his analysis of function is mechanistic [556]. In 1802, the English clergyman Archdeacon William Paley wrote: "... there is precisely the same proof that the eye was created for vision, and that the telescope was created to assist it". William Paley's statement raises the question: does the human body work like a clockwork?

L. Karhausen, *The Fragility of Philosophy of Medicine*, Philosophy and Medicine 147, https://doi.org/10.1007/978-3-031-41633-0_11

Machines are kinds of things that have been built by human beings for their own purposes. The functions of gears and cogs or any other part of a machine are clearly defined and limited. These functions cannot be discovered: we do not need to set up a scientific research project to observe them.

Machines are intentional devices: they have an intentional content; they have a purpose and reflect the intention of the creator. They are constitutively teleological. Clocks are systems in which each element is necessary to achieve the predefined goals for which they were built [557]. A good instrument keeps its promises; a faulty instrument lacks excellence and quality: what makes it good logically takes precedence over what makes it bad.

We define the failure of a machine in syntactic terms, and the failure of an organ in semantic terms. In the first case, the breakdown represents a failure of the logic underlying the machine: it is internal to its mechanism. But in the second case, the failure is contingent on the explanatory model that the physiologist assigns to the organ concerned: it is external to our conventional representation and to the counterfactual nature of physiology.

Indeed, naturalistic normality consists in the fact that the quality of the functions of parts and processes contributes statistically to rigorous and durable products. A good quality machine should have few or no defects.

The function of an organ cannot be reduced to a mechanistic discourse.

11.1 The Teleological Explanation

Aristotle wrote that "nature does nothing without purpose or in vain". He distinguished between efficient and final causes [558]. In one sense, the efficient causes of a thing bring it into existence, while the final causes are its goals or purposes. In another way, teleological explanations—that is, explanations based on ends and final causes—explain the existence of an attribute of a system by showing the positive contribution of that attribute to achieving a preferred state of the system.

The classic function puzzle is how the consequences of a trait can explain why that trait is in fact present.

To a biologist or physician, the activity of the lungs and kidneys is to keep the pH of the blood constant, and the heart contracts to pump blood, which is to assume purposes that can help us understand the natural world.

On the one hand, artefacts are objects made by a designer, so teleological features are the prerogative of human or rational beings; they could not come from organisms lacking intentions and reasoning capacity; they could not arise from unintended and unplanned interactions between mere material bodies.

But on the other hand, in the absence of intentions as in the case of physical events, teleological explanations imply that the present is determined by the future; the heartbeat is explained in relation to blood flow: this would suggest reverse causality, i.e., a philosophical and scientific anathema.

Larry Wright [559] offers the following analysis of functions:

The function of *O* is *F* means

(a) *F* is a consequence (or result) of the presence of *O*, (b) *O* is there because it does *F*.

According to Wright, this definition applies to biology as well as to artefacts; it provides a criterion for distinguishing a function from a mere effect; and it accounts for the normativity of functional ascriptions, so that dysfunction is a natural possibility.

The above raises two sets of questions.

The first question concerns the very nature of the concept of function. Functions, for Wright, are thus natural genera, if natural genera are those that support certain modal implications necessary for biological science.

Functions are family resemblances; multiple, they are related to each other by a series of overlapping similarities in which no single characteristic is common to all: the function of the heart is to pump, the function of the feet is to walk, just as the function of the shape of the nose is to hold a pair of spectacles to the face as Dr Pangloss observed. Because it is a noun, we are led to consider 'function' as an entity with a distinct existence and location.

The second question concerns the perplexing problem of final causes that confronts the philosophy of medicine.

For Larry Wright, the effect explains the cause. He substitutes a causal analysis for a teleological one, and to do this he proposes that a trait has a function because it has been favoured by natural selection. But one does not legitimize teleology as "evolutionarily selected effects" [560] by a genetic fallacy.

"This doctrine of final causes," Spinoza wrote, "turns Nature completely upside down, for it regards as an effect what is in fact a cause, and vice versa." Spinoza reduced explanations by finality to causal explanations [561].

Immanuel Kant argues that "Medical physiology assumes with confidence, and with general approval, that everything in an animal has its utility, and serves some positive purpose" [562]. Kant admits that ends are not observable and are not constitutive principles of reality: "...they are only regulative guides in our judgments and investigations" [563]. He adds: 'The principle of finality... is a heuristic principle for studying the laws of nature, even if we do not wish to use it to explain nature itself' [564].

In this view, the interpretation of functions depends on our cognitive interests [565]. They are projections of our own desires into nature.

But then, is it possible to avoid the classic conundrum of functions mentioned above, namely that the consequences of a feature should explain why that feature is in fact present?

It is John Searle who shows us that functions and their purpose are not, as Boorse would have us believe, natural species, but are a matter of grammar. When we discover the function of the heart, we discover, according to John Searle, how certain causes act to serve certain purposes, but the notion of purpose does not reflect the laws of nature: they do not belong to nature independently of our mind but are relative to our set of values [566]. Functions are always relative to the observer, since they depend on the interests, values, and purposes we attach to things. Functions are never intrinsic to any phenomenon.

On the one hand, Searle argues that functions depend on values. Since values are subjective, it follows that functions are subjective. We talk about a better or worse heart, but never about better or worse stones, unless we attribute a function to them, for example as paperweights. "We anthropomorphize the heart or the kidney as we do the sun or the rain [567, 568]. When we speak of functions," Searle writes, "we speak of those of its causal relations to which we attach some normative significance" [569].

On the other hand, he argues that functions are not natural facts, even though they involve causal statements such as 'the contractions of the heart muscle cause blood to flow' which are perfectly objective and natural.

We say that the function of the heart is to pump blood, just as we say that rivers serve to irrigate the fields, that herbs serve to improve our cooking, that the sun serves to illuminate the surface of the earth. Everything that surrounds and serves the human being has a function: this is the result of an unspoken expectation, which proposes prudential functional models and certain paradigmatic conventional regularities against which sick people or disease entities are evaluated.

Except for the fragments of the world with consciousness, there is no intention, no function, no teleology in the physical or biological world. We can also make objects to perform a certain function, such as chairs, roads, umbrellas, etc. These functions are never intrinsic properties of the physical nature of these objects. These functions are never intrinsic properties of the physical nature of these phenomena: they are assigned by conscious observers, so they are relative to the observer, and therefore external.

When it is impossible to appeal to values, we never speak of functions, for example in the case of malignant tumours or osteoporosis. We discover functions in nature if this is done within the framework of a prior attribution of values, which includes goals or a kind of teleology. If we assume that, for an organism and a species, survival and reproduction have a value, we can state that the function of the heart is to pump blood. If, on the other hand, we do not take survival and reproduction for granted as values, if what we value above all else is death and extinction, then we can say that the purpose of cancer is to hasten death, the purpose of ageing is to hasten death, and the purpose of natural selection is extinction.

In short, when we think of functions, we are referring to relationships to which we attach some normative importance. The causal structure of physiological processes is intrinsic to the organism, but functions are never intrinsic but always relative to an observer.

John Searle did not solve the problem of the origin of functions: he dissolved it into the grammar of medical language.

11.2 The Logic of Functions

Functional descriptions are not predictive since the final object may well be absent. Goal failure, aimlessness, impeding objects or factors are part of reality and partly coextensive with the domain of pathology.

Functional statements describe propensities directed towards a goal with no guarantee of achieving it. A function is not a simple occurrence or sequence of occurrences, as it is not an occurrence but a disposition. It represents a causal power or potential, an ability, a capacity, or a propensity.

Nancy Cartwright writes: "the logic that uses what happens in ideal circumstances to explain what happens in real circumstances is the logic of tendencies or capacities" [570].

Provisions are conditional or hypothetical statements, i.e., statements containing an actual or implied "if": "If *p* then *q*". The antecedent clause p represents the a priori necessary normal conditions in the absence of which the function is not performed: these are the permanent conditions (the physiological context displayed by the whole organism, internal activation conditions, for example, the electrical impulses of the sinus node) or the absence of troublesome environmental or internal conditions (such as heart block). This is to say that the assertability of functional statements does not depend on their actual occurrence, nor on the occurrence of their effect, because functional processes are present intermittently due to the dysfunctions that occur. The attribution of functions does not depend on dated occurrences, but on universal and repeated forms of events, which may or may not be realized. Even if the efficient pumping of blood is a criterion for the proper functioning of the heart, the heart is defective in a significant fraction of cases.

But physiological functions are counterfactual. The function could not have been performed if the necessary factors that constitute it had been absent or if those that hinder it had been present.

Let $Y^i = (y^1 + y^2 + y^3 \ldots + y^n)$ be the set—assuming it is countable—of enabling and activating factors that are necessary and sufficient for the proper performance of a function: these occurring conditions must be jointly present for the function to be truly assigned. The Löwenheim-Skolem theorem in logic indicates that any countable set of sentences that has a pattern, has an infinite countable pattern. In other words, the formulas of predicate logic are only satisfiable in countable domains, namely, the set, assuming it is countable, of enabling and activating factors that are necessary and sufficient for the proper performance of a function: these occurring conditions must be jointly present for the function to be truly assigned [571].

Yet this definition of function takes the no-obstacle clause for granted. Suppose, then, that we can also compile an exhaustive list of all potential hindering factors, disruptive causes or pathological states that could individually cause goal failure: let us call it Xi; the members of the set of hindering factors $X^i = (x^1 \text{ or } x^2 \text{ or } x^3 \ldots \text{ or } x^n)$, if present, are individually sufficient for the failure of the goal.

It follows that if one of the necessary factors is absent or one of the hindering factors is present, the assignment of a functional capacity is subject to cancellation, i.e., the heart does not actually perform its function. A normal function can then be defined as follows:

(1) If the necessary factors Yi are all present and none of the obstacles Xi are present, then the core fulfils its function F.

But propensities are counterfactual properties. To apply to dysfunctions, (1) must be extended to the subjunctive. A dysfunction is then defined as follows:

(2) If the Yi factors were all present and none of the Xi obstacles were present, then the heart would fulfil its function F.

In summary, the function of an organ, as it were, is not only the result it brings, but the result it is supposed to achieve in a way, it still has the same function even if it does not fulfil it.

11.3 Functional Role and Functional Capacity

Functional capacities are ideal capacities stored in physiology textbooks (such as the law of perfect gases or Newton's universal law of gravitation), and which remain true even when functioning abnormally: thus, functional capacities support counterfactuals.

Functional roles, on the other hand, are empirical and factual: they are measured and evaluated in a clinical situation on individuals, or in an epidemiological survey.

A functional capacity could be truly attributed to the system, if and only if it is a priori necessary for the system to achieve its objective, if normal conditions were met and if no impeding factors were present.

Functional capacities are de re, while functional roles are de dicto.

Functional capacities ignore dysfunctions, while dysfunctions represent diminished functional roles: in such cases, the purpose may be absent, but the functional description is still appropriate. Thus, a failing heart has a diminished functional role; and medical care attempts to bring it closer to its functional capacity, to its ideal, i.e., counterfactual, normal physiological function.

11.4 Are Diseases Dysfunctions?

Boorse considers diseases to be an internal state that impairs or limits the ability to function. "Normal functioning is defined in relation to a reference class which is a natural class of organisms of uniform functional design (i.e., within a specific age group and sex), when a process or part (such as an organ) is functioning in a normal way, it makes a statistically typical contribution to the survival and reproduction of the individual whose body contains that process or part." Some deviations from these natural functions may be indifferent or beneficial, but others are not. The latter are diseases [572].

To define a disease, PH. Schwartz mentions an approach requiring dysfunction [573] and for Smart, diseases are alterations of natural functions [574]. For L. Nordenfelt, "disease is identical to the abnormal functioning of the organ or other part" [575].

In fact, dysfunction is not the sum of the characteristics that a disease must have to be called a disease. If dysfunction were a defining characteristic, a process would not be a disease if it did not have dysfunction.

On the other hand, Reznek denies that dysfunction is a necessary condition for disease: an abnormal function is not necessarily a pathological function, so it cannot be either manifest or synonymous with a pathological process [576]. An injury, a bone fracture, is not a process but an event and does not run counter to physiological principles. Ventricular extrasystoles are dysfunctions but most of them do not reflect a disease. Finally, what links disease and dysfunction is a matter of discovery, not of some stipulative definition.

As another example, half of heart failure patients have a normal preserved ejection fraction (HFpEF): the percentage of the volume of blood ejected from the left ventricle with each heartbeat divided by the volume of blood when the left ventricle is at maximum filling is normal.

For all these reasons, disease is one thing and dysfunction is another.

11.5 Dysfunction

Medicine navigates between the conventions of physiology and the characteristics of pathology. It is concerned with deviations or alterations from these ideal and counterfactual norms of functioning in situations where these norms are assumed to decline or no longer apply.

In the case of severe cardiac arrhythmia or ventricular arrest, the heart is unable to maintain its workload, but its function remains that of sending blood to the lungs and the rest of the body.

When the goal is not achieved, we use the following subjunctive conditional:

(3) If some of the necessary factors Y, $Y^i = (y^1 + y^2 + y^3 \ldots + y^n)$ had been absent or if only one obstacle $X^i = (x^1$ or x^2 or x^3 ... or $x^{n)}$ had been present, then the function F would not have occurred.

Functions may not be in regular working order either because they function excessively or insufficiently (hyper- and hypothyroidism), or because their output deviates strongly from physiological norms and is detrimental to the organism (autoimmune diseases, hallucinations). A function may also be prevented from functioning because of resistance to peripheral signals (insulin resistance in type II diabetes, leptin resistance, which is common in obesity, resistance to blood flow in hypertensive vascular disease).

Goal failure implies that a certain goal can be achieved under physiological circumstances [577, 578]. The role of a blind eye is still to see. But the degree to which this goal is achieved, or the failure of expectation, measures the functional capacity of the eye. Functions and dysfunctions have no residence, as dysfunctions, in the biological world, and must simply be adopted for heuristic and pragmatic reasons to undertake a medical investigation [579].

Physiology texts separate the inseparables, i.e., functions from dysfunctions and take sides against the latter. Much that is inappropriate or disfigures clear objectives or defined notions of function is conveniently dumped into the category of pathology. Empirically, functions are confused with dysfunctions, but they are also counterfactually defined, and grammatically separated from them. Functions, Austin would have said, are 'constitutionally iffy'.

To cite another example, angiotensin is a substance that belongs to a class of proteins involved in the regulation of blood pressure. What is its function? It stimulates the release of aldosterone from the adrenal cortex, a hormone that causes an increase in blood pressure. In addition, angiotensin causes vasoconstriction or narrowing of the small blood vessels, which leads to an increase in blood pressure. In cases of severe bleeding, its role is to reduce blood and fluid loss by constricting the vessels and promoting blood clotting.

But that's not all. Angiotensin can also cause considerable long-term damage: as well as increasing blood pressure, it promotes the development of atherosclerotic plaques in the arteries, helps to cause these plaques to rupture, and increases the degree of hypertrophy of the heart muscle after a myocardial infarction; here we have a protein that is unique to the body and has a hormonal function, but which plays an important role in promoting chronic disease. By understanding its mode of action, we therefore divide the effects of angiotensin into those that are useful, which we call its functions, and those that are harmful, which we relegate to pathology.

It follows that the same notion of function, as it were, presupposes the prior notion of dysfunction and that dysfunction delimits the boundaries of function. Conversely, to say that an organ "functions well" is to say first that there is nothing abnormal. The term "function", like "normal", "adapted" or "healthy", is a privative term. It does not emerge on the surface of things but is articulated around a hypothetical subjunctive. Again, *Omnis determinatio est negatio.*

The concept of "function" is born of the illusory idea that behind imperfection lies the general idea of perfection. "Normal" is the default position and means nothing other than "not abnormal". This is in sharp contrast to the case of artefacts: being defective for a machine is privative, so that normality here is logically prior. A good watch logically takes precedence over a defective watch.

Considering the above, it seems that abnormal functioning is foundational; it has the first word and is logically prior to normal functioning. We look for causal explanations for malfunctions, not for functions. When we think of one process as impeding another process, the second is a function: the impediment delimits the function. If we accept that sight depends on the eye, the contrast class of the defective vision defines the function of the eye. It follows that the functions of an organ are not considered normal by virtue of some beneficial effect, but because they do not cause harm. Normal functions play a mere permissive role: they are a posteriori necessary but not sufficient conditions for health and well-being. The silences of physiology on clinical reality tell us much more about what we should avoid than about what we seek. Only rules that hold can be broken. There is no obstacle where there is no function. You must have goals to fail to achieve them. Hindering factors are therefore constitutive of the concept of "function".

To conclude: only abnormal functions or dysfunctions, their degrees and nuances are on the surface of things, while functions are hypothetical and paradigmatic medical standards. It is therefore not surprising that physiological research, which claims to be the study of "normal" functions, has since Claude Bernard proceeded by studying highly abnormal conditions, and that functional attributions have often been tested in experimental medicine by adding and removing organs, or by setting up extreme pathological situations, such as animals deprived of thyroid or pancreas, or by studying patients missing large parts of the brain.

The physiologist Homer Smith observed long ago that defining normal as the relationship between design and function is not very useful: "If it is normal for an intact wheel to run according to its design, is it not also normal for a broken wheel not to run according to its design? "Is it not normal for a diabetic to have glycosuria, for a moron to be exactly what he is, for a malignant tumour to do exactly what a malignant tumour does, for a schizophrenic to behave like a schizophrenic?" [580].

Chapter 12
Treatment, Placebos and Nocebos

The best practitioners give to their patients the least medicine
Frederick Saunders

Abstract Treatment in medicine is a medical intervention that can be performative, intentional, emotional, hortatory, or persuasive, which assumes patient compliance. A treatment may be efficient or effective. Abortion, or euthanasia, even without request may sometimes be therapeutic options. Most treatments have undesirable side-effects. Placebos and nocebos are part of the meaning of therapeutic procedures.

Keywords Treatment · Placebos · Nocebos · Efficiency & effectiveness · Abortion · Euthanasia · Magic bullets

The term "treatment" is used in two different ways. On the one hand, in our medical texts, the term 'treatment' is used in a cognitive and referential mode, in which case the scientific language is out of this world: it refers to an up-to-date medical doctrine on the various aspects of the management of a given condition.

On the other hand, the clinician's language can also be at a different performative, intentional, emotional, hortatory, or persuasive: it is internal to the world, as a set of processes interacting with the world. In this view, utterances are not only used to say things, to report states of affairs, but rather to actively do things, i.e., to perform an act, like the words "I prescribe" or like a bedside dialogue [581].

During the First World War, Wittgenstein had carried out research into the physiology of shock [582]. In 1941, eager to contribute to the war effort, Wittgenstein began working at Guy's Hospital in London as a dispensary porter. Soon after his arrival, he became a pharmacy technician, making Lassar's ointment.

He left Guy's Hospital in 1943 to work with Dr R.T. Grant who had studied at the hospital. Grant who had been studying 'wound shock' at Guy's Hospital. Wittgenstein suggested that the word 'shock' was inappropriate because too many different cases were being diagnosed in this way, making it impossible to assess the value of different treatments. Grant acknowledges that Wittgenstein's influence played an important part in the abandonment of the word 'shock' in his report to the Medical

L. Karhausen, *The Fragility of Philosophy of Medicine*, Philosophy and Medicine 147, https://doi.org/10.1007/978-3-031-41633-0_12

Research Council. Wittgenstein had discussed the issue with Grant and had worked as his laboratory assistant from April 1943 to February 1944.

Wittgenstein was also involved in a research project on the Pulsus Paradoxus, inventing an innovative device for recording pulse pressure.

Had he not thought in 1935 of going to Dublin to study medicine? [583].

While medicine is concerned with treating disease, it is also important to comfort those who are suffering. Indeed, by focusing on the patient's illness, there is a risk of completely abstracting from their suffering, and something valuable could be lost. Wittgenstein emphasized the importance of this second approach in the clinic [584].

These two ways of speaking, semantically and pragmatically, correspond to two modes of relating to the world and to people. These two points of view can be translated in terms of the different oppositions we establish between medical science and medical practice, between what we do and what happens to us, between subject and object, between saying and doing [585].

In short, part of the excess of meaning conveyed by the implicatures of the doctor's discourse comes from his persuasive authority or charisma. The gap between these two functions of language separates the cognitive use of medical language from its performative role, its semantic function from its implicatures, i.e., from medical practice, the personalization of medical care, and public health decisions.

12.1 Efficiency and Effectiveness

There are two ways of expressing the beneficial effect of an intervention: effectiveness and efficiency, depending on whether they are defined and evaluated in a purely descriptive or experimental framework. Both are expressed in terms of probability, i.e., they are depersonalized [586].

Effectiveness, as defined by Archie L. Cochrane, is a measure of the ability of a specific therapeutic regimen to do what it is intended to do in an observational study under ordinary circumstances, i.e., close to what happens in the clinical or public health setting.

Efficacy is a measure of the ability of a specific therapeutic regimen to do what it is designed to do in the experimental setting of a randomized clinical trial (RCT) or a randomized Mendelian trial.

12.2 What Is a Treatment?

A medical intervention ideally seeks to achieve certain ultimate goals such as eradicating or curing a disease, slowing its progression, relieving suffering and other symptoms, preventing disease or injury, recurrence, complications, co-morbidity, or premature death, limiting disability and reducing communicability, restoring functional capacity, as well as providing palliative care for those who cannot be cured. It includes actions such as the administration of medication or other specific measures, such as surgery, physiotherapy, radiotherapy, psychotherapy and lifestyle counselling, assistance, and nursing care in the case of chronic diseases, rehabilitation or re-education, social work, and counselling on the modification of personal behaviour, lifestyle or eating habits. In the case of chronic diseases, treatment should also help patients to live better. This also means that it should—at least as a general principle—focus as much on the patient's environment as on the internal problems specifically inherent in the disease process.

An ideal treatment should fulfil the following conditions:

(0) *Primum non nocere.* "Sometimes it is good medicine to use nothing", wrote Hippocrates (460?–377? BC). Many diseases have a strong tendency to heal with, without or despite medical intervention. Like the restoration of paintings, the first principle of medical care is therapeutic abstention: vigilant monitoring and no treatment are often the best treatment. Any therapeutic decision must be a justified exception to this rule. There is a famous fable by La Fontaine, "*La mouche du coche*", about a fly that, by biting the horse's rump, convinces itself that it is pulling the cart. Practitioners inevitably tend to play the fly in the ointment.

(1) A treatment is a planned *medical intervention.*

(2) It is intended to be *beneficial* even though it may in fact fail to be so, even though Paracelsus (1493?–1541) said: "Only he whose remedies are effective is a physician". It is in the best interest of the patient.

(3) It is based on the conviction, supported by evidence, that it is *effective*, i.e., that its administration will increase the likelihood of improvement of the disease concerned compared to the likelihood of this happening in the absence of intervention.

(4) Being a precautionary act, it should do more good than harm. It should *balance benefit and risk*, and gain and cost. Most treatments have unintended effects, some of which are undesirable. Adverse effects raise the issue of comparative risk: if two treatments are equally effective, the one with less severe and less frequent side effects should be chosen.

(5) In its mode of application, although the disease must be understood as affecting the whole patient, the treatment must be *minimally comprehensive.* In other words, treatment applies to the patient, not the disease. However, well-defined, and curable acute illnesses (such as acute appendicitis or a fracture) in healthy people do not require the kind of meaningful empathic relationships that are required for long-term care in chronic illnesses, in psychiatric syndromes or in the final phase of a terminal illness with a predictable course.

(6) *Compliance* describes the degree to which a patient correctly follows medical advice. It most often refers to adherence to medication or drugs, but it can also apply to other situations such as the use of medical devices, self-care, self-directed exercise, or therapy sessions. Non-compliance is the bane of clinical

medicine and medical investigation. When some say that statins and antidepressants "are not as effective as many people think", they often ignore the clinical reality of non-adherence, which has been established for statins and antidepressants among others [587].
(7) It allows people to die in comfort or with dignity.

Philosophers of medicine have little or no interest in therapeutics [588]. It is true that philosophers who think from their armchairs find themselves embarrassed by the complexity of the forms of life represented by medical interventions. This is probably why they prefer to avoid the subject.

Maël Lemoine in his *Introduction à la philosophie des sciences médicales* devotes no chapter to this subject [589]. As for Anne Fagot-Largeault [590], she limits herself to ethical considerations; or else, they concern a detailed and in-depth analysis of the application of the Bayesian method, which is not without utility, but which is hardly used in the practice of the hospital or private medical clinic. However, it is limited to a formal analysis, but ignores its philosophical aspect (which has been criticized by Nancy Cartwright, one of today's leading philosophers of science) [591]. Her book covers important topics in the history of medicine or medical research but avoids philosophical issues.

12.3 Abortion

Abortion raises a particular problem. It is based on the claim that the fetus has no right to remain in the womb because maintaining its life would require efforts on the part of the woman to which it is not entitled. It is not entitled to such efforts because (i) the efforts are greater than those the woman would be obliged to make to help anyone else. (ii) because deliberately starting to make efforts for someone is not in itself a promise to continue. (iii) in losing life, the fetus only loses what it would not have had anyway without the woman's efforts, so that it is no more unfortunate to have been in the womb and died than if it had never lived at all [592].

Jonathan Glover, Professor of Philosophy at Kings College, London, rejects the idea that human life, as such, or even human consciousness as such, is sacred, and instead defends the theses that it is wrong to destroy a worthwhile human life and to go against the desire of some individuals to continue living. This view implies that consideration of the consequences should play a prominent role in decisions about abortion. Glover is satisfied with this implication and rejects two doctrines, often invoked in these contexts, which would make the link between the morality of an act and its consequences more indirect: the 'double effect', which relies on a distinction between intended and intended consequences, and the doctrine that acts with bad consequences are always worse than omissions with the same consequences; if omissions can be as blameworthy as actions, our failure to save lives can be equated with murder.

Abortion is on the same level as contraception (the difference is in the effects on people other than the fetus or potential fetus). Since the fetus cannot be said to have a desire to continue living, the relevant principle is that of human life worthy of the name. Under this principle, both contraception and abortion are justifiable to avoid the consequences of producing a life not worth living either because the child is unwanted or because it will be severely disabled. However, Glover does not crudely equate physical disability with the absence of a dignified life, and he includes a sensitive discussion of the relationship between the two [593].

12.4 Euthanasia Without a Request

Since the Second World War, no one can write sympathetically about the acceleration of death without being haunted by the Nazi experience.

However, in recent decades there has been an evolution in end-of-life options [594]. Euthanasia is when a doctor voluntarily causes the death of a patient, with the aim of putting an end to suffering deemed unbearable. A distinction is made between active euthanasia, where death is directly caused by the administration of a lethal substance by a doctor, and passive euthanasia, where death is brought about by the cessation of care.

In France, the Leonetti law sets out the rights of patients at the end of life in France. Active euthanasia is prohibited, but so are “unreasonable obstinacy” by the medical profession and “artificial prolongation of life”. Rather than therapeutic obstinacy, the law authorizes the doctor to reduce or stop the treatment of a patient at the end of life, even if this leads to his or her death in the short or long term: passive euthanasia is therefore tolerated in France.

In other words, passive euthanasia consists of washing one’s hands of it, and suspending palliative care, notably infusions and oxygen therapy, i.e., letting a patient die of thirst, hunger, and suffocation.

Jonathan Glover, Professor of Philosophy at Oxford University, has given a wonderful example of how philosophy can illuminate and be illuminated by practical problems. He examines the arguments used to prohibit the killing of others and considers the difficulties posed by advances in modern medicine. When a person has a disease from which he or she has no hope of recovery and which is destined to kill him or her quickly, it is often suggested that medical intervention that goes beyond relieving pain or distress does not save life but prolongs the act of dying. The central question is whether this person has a life worth living? Does this kind of life justify the efforts to preserve it and the effects of this preservation on other people?

In 2002, Belgium passed a law that decriminalizes euthanasia in certain situations. At the patient’s request, a doctor can perform euthanasia if the conditions set out in the law are met. This request is expressed by a capable and conscious patient (current request) or takes the form of an advance declaration (irreversibly unconscious patient).

12.5 The Magic Solution

The German medical scientist Paul Ehrlich (1854–1915), known for his pioneering work in immunology, bacteriology, and chemotherapy, believed that diseases should be cured using a chemically specific therapy, which he compared to "magic bullets" that hit their target and hurt nothing else.

Similarly, each of us tends to believe in the reality of disease entities or the existence of "real" causes, and we are inclined to think that for every condition there must be specific therapeutic remedy. One of the leading philosophers of medicine, Jacob Stegenga, believes that "the metaphor of the bullet...continues to serve as an example for current medical interventions" [595]. The quick fix is the counterpart of the necessary causes. The cure is something that exists, waiting to be discovered, even if it is not yet available, but if we keep looking for it, we will discover it one day. Put your diagnosis in the slot and wait for your treatment ticket to come out of the machine.

Of course, infectious diseases are specific conditions with specific causes. Their discovery has led to a dramatic increase in the healing power of medicine. Vitamin B12 for a patient with pernicious anemia is a miracle solution. Similarly, the development of genomics could bring the next promised medical revolution.

But even here it is a misguided view [596], stemming from the clock analogy whereby we tend to compare disease to a broken clock and disease processes to breakdown in biological congruence. Treatments are rarely precisely targeted, such as ascorbic acid in the case of scurvy. We can conclude with Rudolf Virchow (1821–1902): "From the fundamental error that specific remedies were created for particular diseases arose the idea that the whole course of a disease, or even its different stages, could be annihilated by a single remedy."

Most medical interventions are only partially targeted. They are often accompanied by deleterious and, in the long term, undesirable but hardly avoidable side effects. The choice and development of therapeutic methods aim to reduce the frequency and importance of these side effects. Post-marketing surveillance (PMS) and pharmacovigilance are practices for monitoring the safety of a drug or medical device after it has been placed on the market, and for reporting adverse effects. Toxicity of new agents has often only been discovered after their regular use, as prior detection of adverse reactions can be an intractable problem.

However, we may be reaching a turning point. On the one hand, several new and experimental therapies meet the criteria of the magic bullet, such as CAR-T cell therapy to treat melanoma or certain solid tumours, or long-term gene therapy for children with spinal muscular atrophy. Gene therapies mainly treat diseases.

On the other hand, CRISPR therapy is a way to repair, cure or reverse genetic mutations that cause disease or otherwise shorten life. It offers the possibility, through "in vivo" gene editing, of banishing hereditary diseases from the gene pool. The dilemma facing the scientific community is ethical, with unintended consequences or 'off-target effects'. Where should the line be drawn between eliminating human suffering and manipulating the genetic heritage of future generations?

12.6 Placebos and Meaning

Michel de Montaigne observed: "There are men on whom the mere sight of medicine is operative". In clinical care, a placebo is a therapeutic procedure (or component thereof) administered by a caregiver or used by a patient for a medical condition (disease, disability, or symptom) for which it is biomedically inert, ineffective, and inefficient. More specifically, a placebo "is any therapy knowingly or unknowingly prescribed by a healer, or used by laypeople, for its therapeutic effect on a symptom or disease, but which is ineffective or not specifically effective for the symptom or disorder being treated [597].

Words, gestures, expressions, and placebos only come to life within a language game, a culture, or a way of life, but also according to the context. If a placebo means something, then it means something to someone. Its meaning is not an objective property of the placebo, as are its size and shape. What matters to you depends on how you live (and vice versa), and this shapes your experience. Wittgenstein writes: "The arrow points only in the application that a living being makes of it" [598].

Placebos should have no therapeutic capacity, or at least no specific therapeutic capacity for the condition for which they are targeted: their impact should be limited to a no treatment effect. But this is a theoretical view, which may be true, though rarely so, in narrow experimental settings such as clinical trials where all or most of the potentially interfering variables are held constant. In real clinical care, the issue is more complex: although they have no specific activity of their own, placebos may have some therapeutic effect, namely the "*placebo effect*". If this is the case, then placebos are factors that under the circumstances have a therapeutic effect: they have a causal capacity but no causal role. It follows that the administration of placebos is different from no therapy.

In purely pharmacological terms, there should be no difference between the outcomes of a no-medication group and a placebo group since neither is receiving an effective agent. Despite this, if we conduct a clinical trial with two baseline rates, a placebo group and an untreated reference group, the difference allows us to quantify the placebo effect, i.e., the healing power of the placebo under the given experimental conditions.

First, a placebo is substantive in nature: it is a biologically inert substance or sham intervention that is usually administered voluntarily to the patient, albeit often without the patient's knowledge, with therapeutic intent.

Secondly, the placebo effect is a process of a relational nature: it is the biological impact of belief in a medical treatment; it is extrinsic, contingent, and is not conferred by any intervention, but depends on how other factors are, since these changes could deprive it of its effect. A doctor may well administer, and often does administer, a treatment in the belief that it is effective when it is not; but its placebo effect, when it occurs, may be known or unknown to the prescriber. And our language becomes somewhat unwieldy when we call such treatments 'placebos', meaning that their effectiveness results only from their placebo effect, the 'placebo effect' merging into the 'placebo': it follows that the term 'placebo' is often used when we mean 'placebo effect'.

Many, but not all, psychotherapies, and especially psychoanalysis, result from the placebo effect. Acupuncture relieves back pain, regardless of where the needles are inserted in the body.

Thirdly, almost a quarter of patients taking placebos report adverse effects (the nocebo effect). In some placebo-controlled clinical trials, the incidence of side effects from the nocebo effect may equal or exceed the incidence of side effects seen in patients taking the active drug [599]. The nocebo effect is associated with the expectation of an adverse effect by the person. The placebo effect is based on the tacit assumption "think good, therefore be good", while the nocebo effect assumes "think bad, therefore be bad".

Patients who did not know they were taking a statin started to report muscle pain, real muscle pain, only when they learned they were taking the drug [600]. Despite this, randomized controlled trials in which patients do not know whether they are taking a statin, or a placebo show identical rates of muscle symptoms in the treatment and control groups.

Disclosure of information about potential or hypothetical side effects may contribute to adverse effects. Whether validated or not, whether causally related or not, side effects are usually reported on the package insert. Patients informed about real or fake side effects reported these symptoms three to four times more than patients in a reference group who were not informed about these symptoms. Packaging can set expectations and encourage nocebos.

Placebos may well have no placebo effect, and treatments may, despite the best intentions of the prescriber, and unbeknownst to him or her, have a mere placebo effect. Homeopathy is a treatment, but its effectiveness is zero, which defines its result, if positive, as a placebo effect.

From a logical point of view, treatments and placebos can be interpreted as asymmetrical binary relationships, i.e., they go in one direction only, from provider to receiver. From this point of view, placebos differ from treatments. A treatment is consciously either self-administered or delivered by a third party, whereas cannot be intentionally self-administered: unlike the former, which is a reflexive binary relationship, the intentional administration of placebos is not reflexive.

The placebo effect is a matter of natural meaning. Natural meaning refers to an obvious correlation: clouds are a natural sign of impending rain. Non-natural meanings are either linguistic, i.e., verbal, or non-linguistic, as shown by gestures or conventional signs such as traffic lights.

12.7 The Nature of the Placebo Effect

The property of being a placebo cannot be deduced from the nature of the medicine or the procedure used. Nor is there any transubstantiation necessary for the same glass of mineral water to be an ordinary drink in a bar, or a placebo in a spa. Nor is it appropriate to assume an additive model in which a placebo is an inert substance + factor *X*, where factor *X* is present in the therapeutic alliance and absent without it. In this respect, being a placebo is not a property as it is not inherent to a procedure or substance: the same substance or procedure may or may not be effective depending on the clinical context.

For an intervention to be a placebo in clinical medicine, the physician must either intend it, or his actions, medication or other intervention must unknowingly have a therapeutic effect; but it is the background of the therapeutic alliance or the therapeutic context, which surrounds the vitamin preparation or the sugar pill, that has produced the placebo effect.

The significance of the difference between treatments and placebos is analogous to the difference between Marcel Duchamp's urinal and a real urinal, which he called a 'ready-made'. Duchamp's urinal is no different from a ready-made urinal, in the same way that the latter is different from a urinal of another brand, shape or colour. So, what makes them different?

The treatment and the placebo in a clinical trial look the same to the doctor and the patient. They look identical. What makes them different is that they play a different medical role: although they seem to have everything in common, i.e., they are the same in nature, they belong to two different medical types.

But the most glaring difficulty with placebos and nocebos effects comes from their troublesome consequences in clinical medicine: they blur the boundaries of diagnostic and therapeutic tools and of clinical interpretation. Wittgenstein observes: "You have to ask yourself what is accepted as a criterion for helping a drug. There are several cases. In which cases should we say: 'It is difficult to say whether it has helped'? In which cases should we reject as nonsense the expression: 'Of course, we can never be sure that it was the drug that helped'? [601].

Incidentally, administering a treatment or administering a placebo are logically opposed to each other, even though a given medical intervention refers to at least one of them but may refer to neither. In saying this, a treatment is the logical opposite of a placebo: they are opposites since they cannot both be true, but they can both be false: the patient can improve by spontaneous remission which is independent of either the placebo or the treatment.

12.8 Explaining the Placebo Effect

Are placebos just artefacts or unwanted "noise" in a clinical trial?

The term "placebo" is Latin for "I will please". It was first used in medicine in 1785. A placebo is a fake drug sometimes defined as a "pretend drug". In a way, the placebo is defined by what it is not, i.e., by what makes it different from a treatment.

In fact, the medical literature suggests that placebos produce great subjective and objective improvement in patients with a wide range of clinical conditions, but especially in those affected by pain, although they are probably useful in asthma, osteoarthritis, hypertension, heart attack and mental disorders.

The conventional wisdom is that the placebo effect does not work for specific reasons but rather for psychological reasons: the mere belief that one is receiving an active drug is enough to produce some effect, whether real or not.

Leaving aside cases where placebo effects are illusory, recent research shows that placebo effects are not fictitious procedures but are real and have positive therapeutic potential [602].

Placebo administration shows a clear dose-response relationship. The magnitude of the placebo response is associated with the colour of the placebo pill, its presentation and the type of information given to patients about the pills; high-priced placebos and branded placebos are more effective than low-priced or generic placebos.

In other words, placebo effects are not just in the minds of patients: they have powerful objective effects on physiological function and pathophysiology, although not all conditions are placebo sensitive.

However, the placebo effect is not a single process, but a plurality of family resemblances, with different mechanisms, which may depend on several factors [603]:

1. First, cognitive factors such as meanings and symbolic meanings, attributions, beliefs and desires, anxiety, and rewards, which operate in their socio-cultural context to induce placebo responses. Patients who believe they have undergone active treatment are likely to show significant and persistent improvement in their physical symptoms, compared to those who thought they had been assigned to the placebo group. For example, the direction of the placebo effect coincides with that of the active treatment, the strength of the former is proportional to that of the latter, the reported side effects of the former are often similar, as are the latency periods required for to become active [604].
2. Secondly, placebo effects are not the result of simple mental activity: placebo administration, when effective, gives rise to specific neurobiological pathways. It appears that placebos cause biological changes in the body when the patient feels better in response to their administration. For example, placebos that relieve pain act by releasing the body's natural opioid substances, endorphins; this placebo effect can be either reversed or partially reversed by a drug, naloxone, which counteracts the effect of opiates, or inhibited by a peptide, cholecystokinin (CCK).

Brain imaging techniques (PET, positron emission tomography, and fMRI, functional magnetic resonance) showed that placebo induced brain changes like those observed with opioid drugs, and that they involved correlation with various neural regions (prefrontal, orbitofrontal and insular cortex). Overall, this suggests that placebo acts by altering CCK and endogenous opioid activity [605].

In addition, administering placebos to people with Parkinson's disease resulted in a release of dopamine (which is suppressed in Parkinson's disease) in the striatum of the brain, changes in the basal ganglia, and activation of thalamic neurons that was as great as when they received active drugs. This clearly shows that placebo effects are not mere experimental artefacts.

3. Furthermore, the potential therapeutic effect of clinical attention and the context of the clinical encounter is crucial, such as meaningful doctor-patient interaction and the therapeutic ritual itself. It is thus a psychosocial effect since the words and ritual of the therapeutic intervention can change the chemistry and circuitry of the patient's brain.

Thomas Sydenham (1624–1689) observed that "the arrival of one good clown has a more beneficial influence on the health of a town than that of twenty donkeys laden with medicine". The presence of the doctor is the beginning of the cure, according to an old proverb. It has long been recognized that diagnostic procedures or the simple start of a treatment, even a non-specific one, make a significant proportion of patients feel better.

4. In addition, compliance is important: compliant patients in placebo groups in randomized controlled trials have much better outcomes, including survival, than their non-compliant counterparts [606–609]. Similarly, the desire not to disappoint may reinforce the placebo effect [610]. High compliance is therefore an indication of a better outcome: controlled clinical trials often suggest that unnecessary therapy is effective when given to compliant patients. High compliance by participants in controlled trials reveals a positive attitude marked by the conviction that the treatment will have beneficial effects; combined with the desire not to disappoint, it explains the strengthening of the placebo effect.
5. Expectations, i.e., the expectation of non-voluntary therapeutic responses to pain and depression, play a key role in treatment outcomes in terms of subjective and objective measures of effect [611–613]. They can be modulated to improve therapy. In a trial that studied postoperative pain over several days, the question was whether placebo effects could be used in conjunction with active treatment to reduce overall drug intake.

The investigators used an intravenous saline solution with a routine analgesic. One group was told that the administration was a simple rehydration solution, and another group that it was a potent analgesic.

The patients' intake of analgesics was monitored. Surprisingly, the group that believed the solution helped analgesia took 33% less active analgesics for the same pain control. There was a second group representing the classic double-blind instructions, which followed the same protocol but was instructed "the solution may or may not be a potent analgesic". In this group, patients took 20% less analgesic medication. In summary, changes in instructions and expectations can modulate responses to placebo [614].

6. Physicians' expectations also matter. Research has shown that clinicians' beliefs can alter the therapeutic context and affect placebo effects. In a trial of analgesics, the placebo effect was significantly lower in the group where clinicians believed that no analgesic treatment was being given, when in fact it was, even though patients were unaware of the different and erroneous information given to doctors.

7. The placebo effect may be a classical conditioning effect acting not only on the patient's symptoms and subjective states of pain, nausea or anxiety but also producing powerful biological effects such as processes affecting immune responses. Past experiences, attention and emotions can influence the perception of symptoms by producing a memory of past effects. Prior exposure to an effective treatment reinforces the placebo effects [615].
8. In addition, a persistent misconception about placebos is that they are ineffective if patients know they are receiving them. Results from several studies have shown that open-label placebo treatment, compared to no treatment, resulted, at least in some patients, in surprisingly higher mean global improvement scores, reduced symptom severity scores and adequate relief scores [616].

12.9 Surgery and Placebos

Sham operations may have a much greater placebo effect than drugs.

Two hundred patients with a blocked coronary artery were randomly assigned to undergo real surgery with a stent and a sham operation. There was no difference in how the patients felt six weeks after the operation. Both groups reported less pain and performed well on treadmill tests [617].

Sham surgery refers to a sham surgical procedure that omits the step that is considered therapeutically necessary. The problem is that sham surgery is not really a placebo. It is an invasive procedure with potential scarring or adverse effects.

Sham surgery has shown that many other unnecessary surgical procedures offer no benefit. Take the example of arthroscopic knee surgery for a torn meniscus or degenerative wear and tear, or vertebroplasty for a fractured vertebra, or surgery for subacromial syndrome, which would be as effective as physical therapy, weight loss and exercise.

12.10 The Placebo Effect Is Sometimes Fictitious

In addition to its real healing power, the role of the placebo effect may, in some circumstances, be purely fictitious: it may then consist of various elements:

1. Firstly, *the natural history of the disease*. Excluding confounding factors such as environmental changes, including the treatment environment (a supportive clinical relationship with the patient) or other treatments, when a patient receives a purported treatment and improves, the patient may be better because of the body's natural restorative processes; in the absence of a reference group or comparison, i.e. in the absence of the natural history of the patient's disease in question, this placebo effect requires the a priori assumption that the outcome of no treatment would have been better, whereas most medical conditions have a natural tendency to improve. The success of medical care depends in part or in large part on the natural tendency of most diseases to heal or improve spontaneously.

The use of placebos in clinical trials controls for natural fluctuations in the course of the disease, such as spontaneous recovery. Clinical conditions such as multiple sclerosis or osteoarthritis have a natural history of improvement and deterioration phases that make it difficult to determine whether an improvement should be attributed to a therapeutic intervention. Thus, any therapy may be followed, in the absence of external causal impact, by spontaneous remission.

2. Secondly, *regression to the mean*, i.e., the statistical tendency of selected subjects with extreme values—especially if the measured characteristics are unstable—to be more normal on retest. This problem explains why patients may appear to improve by a simple statistical artefact and in the absence of effective treatment. In this respect, patients seen in research hospitals, where evaluation of medical interventions through clinical trials is usually done, are likely to be sicker than non-referred patients with the same disease. In many of these diseases, a bad period of worsening may be followed by an improvement.
3. There remain common confounding factors such as *observer and subject bias*, i.e., optimistic assessment of the interpretation of the patient's condition by the caregiver or given by the patient himself. Claude Bernard argued that: "A doctor who tries a remedy and cures his patient is inclined to believe that this cure is due to his treatment."

Chapter 13
Is Medical Grammar Counterfactual?

Nothing we do can be unconditionally defended. It can only be attached to something else, which is established. In other words, no reason can be given why one should (or should have) acted thus, except that by acting thus one has produced such and such a state of things, that one must again accept as a goal.

Wittgenstein [618]

Abstract This chapter shows how, since David Hume, scientific hypotheses have not been mere generalisations, but that they call on an additional and necessary element beyond what is purely factual. This is counterfactual reasoning. Medical language in clinical medicine and medical explanation are counterfactual. Physiology is false and counterfactual.

Keywords Normal · Counterfactual

Scientific hypotheses were viewed by David Hume as mere generalizations and as asserting nothing more than a constant conjunction. Is this analysis adequate, and does it require an additional element of necessary connection beyond purely factual uniformity?

However, Hume added: "If the first object had not been, the second would never have existed [...]".

This approach is sometimes called "*truth by emptiness*", which is the assertion of the subjunctive conditional or the counterfactual: "Although there are not As, if there were As, they would all be Bs" A statement S is vacuously true if it resembles the statement $P \rightarrow Q$, where P is known to be false. Statements that can be reduced (with appropriate transformations) to this basic form include the following universally quantified statements:

(x): $P(x) \rightarrow Q(x)$, where it turns out that (x): $\neg P(x)$.

The empty truth most often appears in classical two-truth-value logic. Indeed, if P is false, then $P \rightarrow Q$ will give a vacillating truth in any logic that uses the material

L. Karhausen, *The Fragility of Philosophy of Medicine*, Philosophy and Medicine 147, https://doi.org/10.1007/978-3-031-41633-0_13

conditional (i.e., $P \supset Q$), put if P is a necessary falsity, then it will also give a shaky truth under the strict conditional. This alternative asserts that if something is A, it is B, but the subjunctive conditional asserts the same thing plus the negation of the existence of any A.

Counterfactual reasoning involves thinking about alternative possibilities for the past or consequences of something that are contrary to what happened or could happen. In other words, you imagine the consequences of something that is contrary to what happened or will have happened ("against the facts").

Suppose that ϕ means to be A, and ψ means to be B. Similarly, $\rightarrow$, is the necessity operator of modal logic. So, $\phi \rightarrow \psi$ should be read as 'If it were the case for ϕ to happen, then it would be the case for ψ to happen.

Consider the following:

"If Ariane had suffered from severe dyspnea, Ariane would have been ill".

If Ariane suffered from severe dyspnea and was at an altitude of more than 3500 m, she would not have been sick.

We both have:

$$\phi \rightarrow \psi$$
$$(\phi \wedge \phi') \rightarrow \neg\psi$$

The first is a subjunctive conditional which is true in all possible worlds.

The second is a counterfactual, which is vaguely true since Ariane has never been at altitude.

13.1 What's Normal

"Normal is the thing you hardly ever get. That's why it's normal." [619]

Physiology or anatomy, which are essentially counterfactual, disregard their ontological and conventional origins and therefore appear to be empirically true and to describe natural order regularities. The physiology and fixed life cycles of living organisms are taken for granted: they constitute the neutral reference group. Medical students learn anatomy and physiology before anatomo-pathology and physiopathology. Normative language is thus transformed into indicative language, true or false, and medical thought becomes naturalistic. This is what Broadbent calls the epistemic position which leads to the practical position. Normality, as we have seen, is multiple.

The grammar of physiology as presented in physiology texts is therefore counterfactual. The propositions of physiology are convenient fictions, akin to rules and guidelines, and reflect normal expectations. This privileged status gives them great explanatory power. They are theoretical paradigms and resemble physically impossible constructs such as ideal gases, perfectly rigid bodies, frictionless planes, instantaneous velocity, and bodies moving in a medium completely devoid of resistance. We know perfectly well that there are no ideal gases or perfectly rigid bodies. It's a joke that physicist's model spherical cows to make the equations easy to manipulate. These are limiting constructions or theories since they only approximate what is observed. In this sense, what physiology teaches is a lie. This is reminiscent of Nancy Cartwright's argument that simple physical laws such as the law of gravity are literally wrong.

Functions represent facts only in closed experimental systems or in circumstances defined as normal. They are identified as if they occur in isolation, that is, cut off from ceteris paribus conditions, unlike in the real world where functions act together and interact in a living organism. Contrary to what happens in the case of a car or a vacuum cleaner, if the science of physiology were complete and well written, and no function of an organism were unknown to us, we would still be unable to explain and predict the actual functional behavior of an organism with its composite and intersecting interactions. It follows that physiology, and its functions are literally wrong. His descriptions ignore deviant processes. Physiology is a default position that separates the wheat from the chaff and, according to Immanuel Kant, assumes as an axiom "*that no organ will be found for an end which is not the fittest and best suited for that end*".

Physiological research, which claims to be the study of "normal" functions, proceeds since Claude Bernard in a counterfactual way, by the study of highly abnormal conditions; functional attributions are often demonstrated in experimental medicine by the addition and deletion of organs, or by the establishment of extreme pathological situations, such as animals deprived of thyroid, pancreas or by the study of patients which are missing a large part of the brain.

According to Michael Schaffer, the realist/antirealist debate involves a false dichotomy. The question underlying the debate is not a question of truth or falsity regarding scientific theories. The real question is how real the theories are, that is, how complete they are in terms of representing the world and how close the words they describe are to reality. The real question is how idealized and how close to reality is a given theory, not just whether it is true or false? Therefore, the goals of science, medical science, or psychiatry involve both truth (according to realism) and utility (according to standard forms of antirealism). Many proofs are approximately true, due to inaccuracies in measurements and the like. Medical assertions and actions are governed by the standard of truth at best approximately justified.

The concept of "normal" is therefore neither realistic nor conventional: it corresponds to the way the world of biology and medicine would be, if it were simpler than it is in several respects, and whether the notion of normality was medically real. Nancy Cartwright and more particularly Michael Shaffer have shown that when idealizations are regimented and simplified in counterfactual terms, we see that they bear on the relations between the actual world (that of illness) and the idealized worlds (those of biologico-medical normality) [620].

13.2 The Counterfactual Language of Clinical Medicine

The type of statement—an "if" statement in which the "if" part is false or unrealized—is a counterfactual, or a conditional whose antecedent is false. "If we had periodically done a colonoscopy, he wouldn't have colon cancer" says when did not do colonoscopies.

A very widespread way of understanding counterfactuals uses the notion proposed by David Lewis of possible worlds [621]: a counterfactual is true when the consequent is true in the nearest possible world, that is, a world as close as possible to ours, in which the antecedent is true.

But that's not all. A counterfactual establishes a dependence, causal or not, between separate events that either are facts that take place in the world or that they are related to each other by a relation of ideas, which can be logical, analytical, or mathematical. This world—the collection of all facts—is the real world.

In contrast, a possible world is an unreal world, a world in which one or more things are not as they really are, but as they could have been. David Lewis argued that possible worlds are real, that is, they have an external, mind-independent existence: what is counterfactual in our world is factual in some other world.

In sum, counterfactual reasoning is essential for rational agents. Causal relations, or natural regularities, are fundamentally different from accidental generalizations in scientific explanations because they support counterfactuals. The key element of the explanation answers the questions "if things had been different".

However, methods for analyzing logical truth functionality do not apply to counterfactuals. In verifunctional semantics, the truth value of a complex sentence is determined by the truth values of its parts. Now, the logic of truth functions is inadequate for counterfactuals because there does not exist, by definition, any functional truth connector which simultaneously combines two false sentences to make a true one, and which combines two false sentences to make a true one false. Furthermore, the truth conditions of counterfactuals are context sensitive.

Clinical medical grammar uses terms and statements that relate to physiology or anatomy or normal laboratory values. These references are all false, true out of emptiness, or at least they are not true. The same is true of the references to the standards of the species used by Christopher Boorse.

Dispositional properties, or capabilities, are quite naturally understood in terms of counterfactual assertions. In the life form of clinical medicine, counterfactuality is grammatical.

Rules are central to clinical medicine because actions are constituted as the actions they are, by the rules that apply to them. Obedience to the rules is implicit in practical knowledge of clinical medicine and actions that are seen to lead to the same. Compliance with the rules cannot rely entirely on linguistically codified explicit knowledge, since such explicit knowledge would require additional implicit knowledge of how the rule is to be interpreted.

When we evaluate indicative conditionals, we add *p* to all our current beliefs, make the minimal adjustments necessary to accommodate it, and examine whether still follows.

But when we evaluate subjunctive conditionals, we proceed differently. We first remove from our current beliefs all those whose truth is a causal consequence of *not-p*—and only then we add *p* with minimal adjustments and consider whether q follows. Since we are concerned with the impact that *p* would have, we do not want to reason based on facts that would have been causally altered if *p* had not been realized

- indicative contrary to facts: "*If the person has signs and symptoms of biological negativities, they have a disease, but this is not the case.*"

When we move from the indicative to the subjunctive, we realize that the biological negativities are real objective, empirical and measurable.

- In the subjunctive: "*If the person had presented signs and symptoms of biological negativities, he would have been suffering from a disease*".

What is normal should not be interpreted as an empirical fixed point, but as a range of variations, tolerated in accordance with an earlier theory of the relationship between individual organisms and the populations of which they are members, a fortiori, between organisms. individuals and their environment.

In short, the grammar of clinical medicine is based on anatomical, physiological, or biochemical norms which are essentially counterfactual.

13.3 The Counterfactual Nature of Medical Explanations

But there is another consideration of immediate interest. Stephen Toulmin writes: "I drop a glass on a concrete floor, and it breaks. So what? This event is so unsurprising that it poses no problem to science. If it hadn't broken, it might have sparked a scientific inquiry: "Why not?" Was there a substance in the glass just before it fell that protected it from breaking? Was there something about the angle exactly what it hit on the ground? Or how else can it be explained that it didn't break as expected?" [622]

The need for explanation is now of the form: "Why shouldn't this have happened?"

This parable emphasizes the importance of anomalies, of events that go against our reasonable expectations. What are the types of medical facts that need to be explained? Not all facts or events require an explanation, only some of their aspects. It is certain that not everything that can be observed during an epidemiological investigation or during medical care should be recorded and explained. A physician may wonder why his patient's heartbeat is irregular, not why it is regular, even though he is supposed to note it in the medical record. Medical investigation is concerned with observable features that are either pathological, raise a legitimate question for research, or constitute a matter of concern for medical insight or a challenge to certain beliefs and knowledge. In principle, the genuine matters which call for a medical explanation are deviations, disturbances, anomalies, and irregularities [623].

Should an abnormal state of affairs be defined as abnormal with respect to accepted normative knowledge, with respect to the normal functioning of the species as Boorse would, have it? Admittedly, in medical language, what is called "normal" constitutes the framework of anatomy, physiology, or biochemistry. Newton's first law states that objects that are not subject to any external force will continue to move in the same direction and at the same speed. Physiology is a set of hypothetical functions that serve the style of explanation that, if left unchecked, things will take their "natural" course. It identifies the phenomena that must be explained by contrasting them with the normal course of things, which does not. This is a negative factual situation. Physiology is false and, like normality, it is non-empirical in character, while the phenomena that pertain to medicine are observable and quantifiable.

Therefore, this definition of the normal and natural order is given in negative terms: the absence of evil, suffering, unmanageable anguish, or handicap. If we take this natural order for granted, then we recognize the proper relationship between physiology and pathology [624]. The concepts of health, function or normality are counterfactual in the grammar of medical language.

It follows that the anomalies are not refutations directed against the context in question. Epileptic seizures, for example, are anomalies. The neuroscientist studies in the same way all the neurophysiological processes that take place in the brain. Thus, the neurophysiologist, unlike the clinical neurologist, treats normal and pathological processes on an equal footing. On the other hand, a certain contrast is necessary for a fruitful medical explanation: a doctor could ask the neurobiologist why his patient presents epileptic seizures rather than none. In other words, explanations have a comparative form. And it is the choice of contrast case that partly determines what counts as a successful explanation.

Abnormal phenomena can therefore be explained by comparing them to other self-explanatory events of the same type, which are inherently more normal or more natural [625].

Chapter 14
The Philosophy of Medicine Versus Medicine

Don't think look!

Wittgenstein

Abstract Literature on the philosophy of medicine is characterized by a thirst for generalities. Wittgenstein's remarks on family resemblances are intended as a refutation of this essentialist view of the meaning of general words. Words in medicine are usually vague and lack precision. Sadegh-Zadeh introduced a theory of fuzzy sets; he defines diseases as a resemblance to a prototype since linguists interpreted Roschian prototypes as members of a category.

The fragility of armchair philosophy is frequent, and is due to the confusion between opinions or beliefs and evidence.

Keywords Philosophy of medicine · Vagueness · Diseases as prototypes · Philosophical speculation

The philosophy of medicine, which should be a chapter of the philosophy of science, has the aim and effect of reflecting on medical science, of seeking to identify the meta-scientific notions that it shares with the other sciences, as well as what separates it from these sciences and from biology. It is not without interest to analyze certain aspects of the relationship between philosophy and medical sciences. This relationship is not asymmetrical, because, while philosophy has medicine as its object, medicine is generally not very concerned with philosophy.

The first problem with the philosophy of medical science is its constant need for generalities and that it is essentialist. The second, as discussed above, concerns the logical priority that philosophy gives to diseases. The third raises the question of the imprecision of medical language. Then comes a critique of the fear of models in the medical sciences. The final problem is the place of scientific truth in the philosophy of medicine. It seems that too often it raises questions about philosophy and medicine, rather than about the philosophy of medicine.

L. Karhausen, *The Fragility of Philosophy of Medicine*, Philosophy and Medicine 147, https://doi.org/10.1007/978-3-031-41633-0_14

14.1 A Thirst for Generalities

Wittgenstein writes: "*The tendency to look for something common to all entities that we commonly subsume under a general term—... The idea that a general concept is a property common to its cases is related to other primitive and overly simple ideas about the structure of language. It is comparable to the idea that properties are ingredients of things that have those properties*" [626]. "*Instead of 'thirst for generalities', I might as well have said 'disdainful attitude towards particular cases*" [627].

One of the sources of this need is the idea that there must be something in common in all the entities we group under the general term of disease, health, function, etc. We assume that there must always be a 'thing' to which each noun corresponds, and which gives meaning to the term in question. This image of the noun as a necessary correspondent to objects has held such sway that when philosophers have failed to find a material or tangible thing to which the noun in question might correspond, they have often succumbed to the temptation to posit theoretically postulated and purely hypothetical 'processes', 'states' or 'things' [628].

Wittgenstein writes: "*An image holds us captive. And we cannot get out of it because it is in our language and language seems to repeat it inexorably". It is this consideration—that an image we may have of the essence of something, or of the way things "must" be, implies that we look at things in such a way that our fixed idea is constantly reinforced—that stands in the way of "an examination of details in philosophy*" [629].

If we move away from nouns in general to focus on the concepts of 'thinking', 'growing old', 'being sick' or 'understanding', we can see how the same prejudice might be what has led many philosophers to assume that these terms correspond to univocal processes.

Wittgenstein's remarks on family resemblances are intended as a refutation of a particular view of the meaning of general words, namely the essentialist view that all entities subsumed under a general word have something in common by virtue of which they are so subsumed.

Do we need the concept of disease? Maël Lemoine and Elodie Giroux raise this question. The answer is in the question. Diseases are clinical and biological processes that have their nosography. On the other hand, disease is a term that belongs to the grammar of medical language and thus plays a role in the organization of medical knowledge; the use of a term does not necessarily mean that it designates a real entity, but its meaning is to be found in the use made of it. The disease is then an example of family resemblances with the accompanying notions of causes, prognosis, prevention, and treatment.

It is defined by a quorum of all diseases. Diseases are life forms, some are acute, some are chronic, some are genetic, some like infectious diseases are defined by a single cause, and they are related to each other by similarities, and some are fictitious.

Wittgenstein, addressing the belief that words are used according to strict rules, said:

> *Do not say: there must be something in common but look and see if there is anything in common... but similarities, relationships, and a whole series of these.*" [630]

> *Not only do we not think about the rules of language—the definitions, etc.—but we also think about how to define them.—not only do we not think about the rules of language—definitions, etc.—when we use language, but when we are asked to give such rules, in most cases we are not able to do so. We are unable to clearly circumscribe the concepts we use, not because we do not know their true definitions, but because there is no true 'definition' for them. To assume that there must be, would be like assuming that when children play ball, they are playing a game according to strict rules.* [631]

Our words are like blurred images, a series of interconnected uses, all bound together by something ambiguous and ineffable; there is an inevitable vagueness that accompanies them.

For Wittgenstein, strict definitions are offered only for their own sake—as if they were a law of language. For Wittgensteinians, this is a terrible confusion that annoys them. Indeed, the idea of 'definition' is thrown at us as if it were a legal matter, and we feel that the matter is out of control. Wittgenstein writes: "*A philosophically perplexed man sees a law in the way a word is used, and, in trying to apply this law consistently, he comes across cases where it leads to paradoxical results*" [632]. For Wittgenstein, there is no question of belief here, there is no crusade for what should or should not be a disease.

Moreover, if there is disagreement about such concepts, each author is merely stating the view he or she favours. And the dissenters merely reveal how they prefer to express themselves on the set of concepts in question. The central question is whether the speech act works, and if so, what it says. The point is that meaning is produced through successful use. Wittgenstein writes: "*The meaning of a word is a kind of use of it*" [633]. This view is action-centered: language is what it does. The key is that it is result-oriented. Only the ends of successful communication matter.

And this raises an interesting question: is there ever anything central or common to the uses of ordinary words? If meaning is a usage, there are no rules for it: intelligibility is a natural phenomenon, and we cannot create rules or structures that invalidate it.

When an epidemiologist, a clinician or a philosopher uses the term risk, they are not thinking of all the considerations mentioned by Elodie Giroux, and these clearly indicate that they are not universals. These different approaches represent "different ways of thinking" [634].

14.2 The Vagueness of Medical Terms

The multiplicity of aspects in which a word can be vague—what Wittgenstein calls *fuzzy concepts* [635]—is a pervasive feature of language that affects even the most scientific terms. It is often very difficult to define a word in the medical sciences where the lack of precision creates areas of indeterminacy. The fact that many words are used in medicine without a willingness to explain their meaning is like saying that "*the light from my work lamp is not a real light, because it has no clear boundary*" [636].

For an expression to be true or false, it must have a meaning. It does not follow, according to Wittgenstein, from the fact that an expression does not have a precise meaning that it is devoid of meaning. What he rejects is not the connection between having a meaning and being true or false, but that the meaning must necessarily be precise [637].

The polar terms are obvious examples: easy, difficult; painful, painless; harmful, harmless; normal, abnormal. Each of these gradually merges into the other and there is no point at which you can draw the line and say: "at this point the clinical situation ceases to be normal and begins to be abnormal". This kind of blurring is quite simple: there is a line or axis at one end of which words are applicable, at the other end of which they are inapplicable.

But what if there is not one line, but several lines, all of which intersect?

There may be several criteria for the use of a word, as in the case of risk or risk factor. A word can have a multiplicity of meanings, but each meaning can have a precise criterion for its application: this is not vagueness. In this case, the word lacks precision because there is no defined set of conditions governing its application. There is no set of conditions each of which is necessary and together sufficient for the application of the word.

Wittgenstein writes: "*But is a concept with fuzzy edges really a concept?—Is a photograph that lacks sharpness really an image of someone? Is it even always an advantage to replace an unsharp image with a sharp one? Isn't the unsharp image just what we need*? [638].

This is where family resemblances come in.

We find a set of characteristics associated with, for example, the word 'disease', not all of which need to be present; in fact, any one of them may be absent—in which case the characteristic is not determinant—and the object will always be a disease if all, most, or some of the other characteristics are present. Moreover, diseases are moving targets with their co-morbidity, and difficult to identify because they change rapidly. The nosologies themselves are plural and each one depends on the use made of it, clinical, preventive, administrative etc.

What sense, then, can be made of debates about the ontology of nosological entities and whether they represent natural species? The classification of natural kinds reflects a problem of our own making, namely our interest in explanation, at least as much as it reflects the actual structure of the world.

Hacking reminds us that there are very few words in everyday language that refer to natural species [639]. Philosophers of biology are far from convinced that species are categories, let alone natural categories. Biological taxonomy, like medical nosography, is a mess [640].

Dupré believes that there are many real similarities and differences in nature, which are logically distinct from our thoughts and beliefs about them, but they generally cannot be 'nested' within each other, and they often overlap. No classification system is primary, fundamental, or privileged [641].

And often there is no definite number of features that make up the set, or we cannot be sure that there are. Not only is it impossible to apply the word by finding the percentage of characteristics that constitute a quorum, but we cannot settle on a defined number of characteristics as the set. This is the case for most psychiatric disorders for which there is no defined set of characteristics to choose from.

Some features are not simply absent or present, but present to varying degrees, and the greater the degree of presence of the feature, the more weight it carries in qualifying the thing in question as a disease. Often it is not possible to state in quantitative terms what weight is added by the degree of presence of the characteristic; one can only say, vaguely, "the more the characteristic is present, the more confidently we can say it is a disease".

Moreover, we cannot foresee all the possible circumstances which, if they arose, would lead us to doubt whether the word is applicable or not.

It should be added that when we define words by using other words, these other words are usually themselves vague. We may define a given disease by characteristics A, B and C, but we may not know exactly what the possession of these characteristics is. The same vagueness that we find in the original term is likely to reappear in the terms we use to define it.

Wittgenstein then introduces two antithetical terms which he illustrates with a medical example. How, for example, does a doctor decide that his patient has pulmonary tuberculosis? He decides this either by *criteria* or by *symptoms*. If the patient has significant lung lesions and his sputum contains Koch's bacillus, this is a "criterion" for tuberculosis. But if, on the contrary, his sputum does not contain Koch's bacillus, his pulmonary lesions may give us a "symptom", i.e., a phenomenon which experience has taught us may coincide, in one way or another, with the phenomenon which is the criterion of our definition [642]. Symptoms are contingent, whereas criteria are a priori.

Moreover, it is a mistake to believe that there is "an indefinite possibility of improving accuracy" [643].

14.3 J Sadegh-Zadeh and Fuzzy Logic

The words of our natural language are inherently vague, and since this means that a word contains more than can be made explicit in a definition, we are led to conclude that there is precision in vagueness since our vague concepts are implicitly understood by native speakers.

Wittgenstein focused on a type of vagueness that is implied by his theory of meaning: there are several independently sufficient conditions for the application of words, not just one, common property shared by the subsumed objects [644].

In this situation, a definition becomes problematic. It cannot specify a common property; it cannot be a generalization; it can only describe a sample. Wittgenstein did not spend much time analyzing the nature of definition, but only its absence in natural language. He argues that definition appears long after we can use our words. "We speak, say things, and only later can we form a picture of their life [645].

In *Tractatus Logico Philosophicus* 3.315, Wittgenstein introduces the notion of a *logical prototype*. He writes that if we were to convert into variables all the signs of a proposition whose meaning depends on an arbitrary agreement, then there will be a class of propositions that are all values of the resulting variable proposition. This class will not depend on any agreement but only on the nature of the proposition. It will correspond, he says, to a logical form, and he refers to it as a logical prototype. In 5.522, he says that pointing to a logical prototype is one of the things that is peculiar to the symbolism of generality.

Proposition 3.24 says that generality notation contains a *prototype*. Proposition 4.0411 considers various ways of expressing generality in logical notation and rejects each of them on the grounds that they lack the necessary mathematical multiplicity. This refers to 4.04, which tells us that a proposition must contain as many things to be differentiated as there are things in the situation the proposition represents. In 5.131, he suggests that no sign of generality is needed, because the symbol "(x) fx" already contains generality. That is, in this context, x already implies that, whatever x is, it is true that fx. And generality is implicit in this "whatever". We do not need to add notation to specify that there is generality here. Indeed, 4.0411 implies that it is impossible to do so.

Wittgenstein's theory of *categories* holds that categories are not discrete and absolute but rather fuzzy-edged and contingent—upon the context/purpose of their use. Cognitive psychology, overwhelmed by Wittgenstein's research on family resemblances, has thus supported the idea of choosing a sample object to serve as a paradigm case.

Eleanor Rosch, a professor of psychology at the University of California, has conducted investigations into our ability to determine class membership [646]. Classes are loosely defined, and *membership is by degrees*. We operate with *prototypes* in mind when we use a word (what Wittgenstein calls a schema [647]). A prototype is an object that most clearly identifies a concept, an object that has the greatest number of characteristic features: a disease for medicine, or a religion for Catholicism. The existence of these prototypes gives the illusion of a defining feature, but their role is not to give a clear definition. Rather, they serve, according to Eleanor Rosch, as practical tools of synthesis. Indeed, they give the appearance of a definition to what is essentially a vague concept. They represent categories as norms or as a set of typical exemplars. Thus, when we think of horses, refrigerators, and policemen in Paris, we retain a representation of one or more 'normal members' of these categories.

By identifying prototypes with attested meanings, cognitive linguists interpreted *Roschian prototypes as members of a category*. It was legitimate to do so insofar as Rosch explicitly invited this interpretation. However, Rosch warned against this interpretation, referring to prototypes as "grammatical fictions" resulting from the reification of typicality judgements.

The German physician and philosopher Kazem Sadegh-Zadeh has investigated which human and biological situations can be held as probable diseases and which are prototypes. In this respect, the notions of health, illness and disease are usually subject to fuzzy theoretical analysis and present themselves as non-Aristotelian concepts that violate the basic principles of classical logic [648].

Lotfi Zadeh as well as Max Black [649],extended the work of Wittgenstein and shared the latter's view of the vagueness of our concepts. In 1965 Zadeh developed a formal apparatus to deal with this issue. He is the founder of *fuzzy logic*, which is widely used in several fields of computer science. In classical logic, a proposition is either true (1) or false (0). Zadeh proposes to use instead a degree of truth, a number that can go from 0 (for false) to 1 (for true) [650].

Zadeh presents a sketch of a theory of the similarity of disease prototypes and proceeds in three steps [651].

1. He rightly criticizes what he calls the "classical concepts" according to which it is accepted that a category is defined by a set of essential characteristics that are both necessary and sufficient for its application. This is because most concepts that are used in everyday life or in various human activities—except for mathematics—are vague, a remark that originates with Wittgenstein [652, 653].

Moreover, he mistakenly attributes this traditional style of thinking to Aristotle [654]: in fact, Aristotle (in his analysis of the polysemy of the concept of "in") is, on the contrary, the originator of the movement of thought "from Aristotle to Wittgenstein" [655], which deals with categories whose members do not necessarily possess common features by virtue of which they fall into that category.

2. In a second and legitimate step, Sadegh-Zadeh explains that the reason for the difficulties in defining illness is that "*there are no properties that can establish the sick being that recur uniformly in all clinical entities to construct an indisputable concept of illness.*" Instead of the old postulate of commonality, he suggests the Wiittgensteinian postulate of resemblance or similarity among all, a concept, that of family resemblances, proposed and developed since the 1930s by Wittgenstein.

14.4 Diseases as Prototypes

In a third and more dubious step, Sadegh-Zadeh introduces the idea of *disease as a resemblance to a prototype*, an idea he borrows from the research of Eleanor Rosch. He then introduces the mathematical theory of fuzzy sets and defines disease as a resemblance to a prototype. The category of diseases is structured around several prototypes from which the inclusion of sub-categories such as infectious diseases, genetic diseases and so on, is organized.

It is hard to see the point of the questions that Sadegh-Zadeh seeks to answer, as they had found their solution in Wittgenstein's notion of family resemblances: there is no indication that Wittgenstein would have approved of these modes of formalizing his work, whether there should be accuracy in imprecision, or whether we can be satisfied with vague imprecision [656]. The vagueness of certain concepts is not provisional but is a feature of logical particularity [657]. If one talks about playing chess, or the violin, or mind games, one hardly needs prototypes to understand what it is all about.

What Sadegh-Zadeh proposes is a brilliant exercise in philosophical speculation, the benefit of which is hard to see. Do health professionals have a prototype concept of disease? Have the prototypes been applied, and if so, by whom? The statement that "disease is a prototype concept" is a testable empirical hypothesis. Therefore, a study was conducted to test the hypothesis that health professionals have a prototype concept of disease. The answer was 'no' [658].

Clinicians, epidemiologists, and health services manipulate, create, destroy, divide, or modify diseases. Sadegh-Zadeh's reflections illustrate the exile in which the philosophy of medicine is sometimes exercised, far, far away from medical realities.

Furthermore, according to Lilienfeld and Marino, it is in principle impossible to explicitly define mental disorder, because disorder is a mental construct that has no clear demarcation point in the real world and no criterion-based attributes. They propose that mental disorders are best conceived as Roschian concepts, which are mental constructs typically used to categorize entities in the natural environment and which are characterized by fuzzy boundaries and the absence of defining features [659].

14.5 Models and Their Fragility

Paul Thompson, professor of philosophy at the University of Toronto, describes the construction and use of models and theories in medical science. He distinguishes the explanatory power of models and theories from the kind of narrow information obtained from randomized clinical trials, because, without an account of the dynamics provided by an appeal to theory, such a trial provides at best evidence for an isolated causal claim [660]. Models and theories involve many variables and equations and are usually broken down into sub-models that describe sub-systems. Theories support counterfactuals and can be used to explain, predict, and manipulate nature.

Such models are ubiquitous in medical science. What is surprising, writes Thompson, is the lack of attention paid to this fact in medicine.

This of course seems philosophically regrettable. The history of physics is a succession of models and theories. In chemistry, biology and astronomy, the development of theories and models is an integral part of science. Not in medicine, except for Pasteur's germ theory.

Why is this so?

Thompson believes that the origins of medicine are more empirical and applied. Clinical practice and medical research have been inextricably intertwined, with theorization taking a back seat. Furthermore, he also attributes this neglect to the minimal relationship between philosophers and the medical professions. The epistemological, metaphysical, and logical aspects of medicine have been neglected and have been submerged over the last 40 years by a fascination with ethical issues.

What are we to make of this critique of Thompson?

According to the constructive empiricism of the Canadian philosopher Baas van Fraassen, we should never believe in the truth of a theory that goes beyond observable phenomena. At most, we should believe that such a theory is 'empirically adequate', that is, that it is correct in what it says about the observable part of the world [661].

Nancy Cartwright states that we use models to predict and navigate the world: they are shortcut labels for the powers and our practices for using them. Any modality is only in the model, in our representation of words, not in the world itself [662].

14.6 Medical Truths and Philosophical Speculation

The debates that are the subject of the philosophy of medicine, for example on whether diseases are natural phenomena, consist of comparing the opinions of different renowned authors.

Everyone, writes Patrick Monahan, is entitled to his own opinion, but not to his own facts. There seems to be a tendency to evaluate information according to its conclusion rather than the validity of the evidence. As a result, the authors do not make a clear distinction between convictions, opinions or beliefs and factual evidence.

For example, the place occupied by Canguilhem in the philosophy of medical science is quite surprising because his writings on medicine are teeming with serious medical errors, such as his advice not to treat arterial hypertension which constitutes for him a new way of life; he criticizes the generalized practices of vaccination which are, again according to him, likely to cause the appearance of microbes more resistant to vaccines, which is false; as for hemophilia, it is not a disease, but an anomaly: "it is nothing, as long as there is no trauma" he writes; and again as his misunderstanding of the new and revolutionary notion of "stress" introduced by Hans Selye. He defends his ideas through a cherry-picking process which consists of supporting his theses with selected references and generally of dubious quality, without citing those who would refute them [663].

Canguilhem, it seems, also commits philosophical errors when he speaks of the normative power of all living beings, normative power which consists in valuing positively or negatively, as attractive, or repulsive, elements of the environment or states of the organism, not by a decision of the individual, but by its biological functions themselves. However, in philosophy, norms are prescriptive, because they do not describe how reality is, but how it should be. They are therefore neither true nor false, but they can be correct or incorrect.

In one of the best books on the philosophy of medicine, the philosopher of science Mario Bunge concludes that "the extravagant view of disease" presented to us by Canguilhem "confuses the normative and descriptive concepts of normality, privileges the former and concludes that illnesses are social deviations, therefore matters of concern in some societies and periods but not in others. It would be the same for health; it would simply be a different social norm... Therefore, medicine would be a "normative project"—just like politics and law" [664].

Recall that Wittgenstein said that there are no norms in nature. Incidentally, this error is called naturalist paralogism, a logical error denounced in 1903 by G.E. Moore and which consists in confusing a normative judgment with a factual judgment: a living organism cannot be mistaken because there is no room for standards of behavior.

Canguilhem thus amalgamates the descriptive with the prescriptive

He makes another mistake when he writes that "Disease arises when the organism is so modified that it comes to catastrophic reactions in its own environment. This is because "...an anomaly, a variation on a specific theme, only becomes pathological in its relationship with a living environment and a way of life..." [665].

What is the relationship between organism and environment that makes pathological osteoarthritis, malignant tumors, amyotrophic lateral sclerosis, genetic anomalies, or trisomy 21? A pathological process is generally internal to the organism and is determined as pathological in and of itself, and independently of the environment, even if the latter is likely to improve or aggravate the symptoms of the disease.

Finally, Canguilhem criticizes medicine and doctors "as regards the abandonment of their vocation to heal in favor of regulated tasks of screening, treatment and controls. » ... « Modern therapy seems to have lost sight of any natural norm of organic life. In this, he rejects preventive medicine.

Canguilhem manifests a nostalgia for Lamarck's evolutionary thought that no one accepts anymore, which leads him to take positions that are aberrant to say the least. He enthusiastically devotes more than a page to the neo-Lamarckian theories of Lyssenko (1898–1976), of which Jacques Monod wrote "that this is the most heartbreaking episode in the whole history of science", and which Jean Rostand described as "delirium based on doctrinal intoxication" or even, according to the historian of science Denis Buican, "an episode worthy of the darkest periods of the Middle Ages. Les surpassant même. » Lyssenko had received the Stalin Prize and was named a Hero of the USSR. Those who knew him—Julian Huxley and Professor Herrmann Muller—observed his profound ignorance of biology; he was arrogant, bigoted, illiterate, and paranoid. Many Russian geneticists who rejected Lamarckism were sent to the gulag, or more simply disappeared [666].

Wittgenstein observed: "*Don't think, look! But everything happens as if a certain philosophy in the bedroom is looking away to avoid confronting these errors or these scientific and philosophical absurdities.*"

All in all, philosophers are sometimes not or little or not at all concerned with the reality and truth of medical knowledge. Here we touch closely on the divorce that separates medicine from the philosophy of medicine.

While medical knowledge proceeds by a *bottom-up* strategy, philosophers follow a *top-down* approach. They seek to confirm, or sometimes invalidate, a set of premises that serve as their starting point. This approach is based on a need for consistency which seems necessary to them. Faced with the real or apparent disorder of the exponential and heterogeneous explosion of medical knowledge, they strive to recognize unified problems and identify patterns of logic of continuity.

Maël Lemoine's wonderful little book on the philosophy of medical science clearly highlights the content of this discipline while revealing its extreme limits.

The philosophy of medical science is the subject of endless debate, and the different opinions which the authors take as incompatible with each other are often, despite the distinctions which oppose them, all valid. These are often reviews of the medical or philosophical literature which are not devoid of interest, and which deal with certain conceptual problems. However, we rarely or exceptionally see here what has made the creativity of philosophy from Socrates and Plato to the present day. The philosophers of medicine represent a kind of international club of brilliant and endogamous intellectuals, who tend to dialogue and debate among themselves about medical sciences, without being too interested in them, and, often, in the ignorance of the philosophy of science and the role that epistemology, metaphysics and formal logic play in it [667]. These authors are interested both in certain aspects of medicine as well as in the varied and often conflicting opinions of their colleagues. They analyze, compare, categorize, and discuss the ideas and doctrines of certain thought leaders, and the differences that distinguish them. The books of medicine serve as an object of reflection for them, so that it is a matter of medicine in a can, and of *armchair philosophy.*

Philosophy, Wittgenstein said, begins when language goes on a journey.

However, the practice of medicine and that of public health are so closely linked that a philosophical analysis which bears exclusively on the first often remains on the surface of things and is inevitably of great philosophical poverty. It is likely to be a passing fad and one that will last until a new generation of philosophers broaden the horizons of the discipline so that it fits into the philosophy of science of which it should be a chapter.

In a preface to the works of Hippocrates published in Paris in 1697, we can read the following: "*The Philosophical Doctors were content with theory and did not descend to practice and experiments, where they practiced only rarely*" [668].

Chapter 15
To Conclude

Don't think look!

Wittgenstein

Abstract Philosophy of medicine is a chapter of philosophy of science. There are two different approaches: philosophy *and* medicine, or philosophy *of* medicine. I chose the second one.

But is there unity or disunity in sciences? Whatever the case, medicine is both a science and a technique, a praxology.

Science is based on the relationship between language and reality, but does reality precede language or vice versa?

The philosophy of medical science is a chapter of the philosophy of science. But it is also exercised in the tradition of analytic and postanalytic philosophy.

This book seeks a new approach to the philosophy of medicine. It remains as close as possible to the medical clinic and public health. It proceeds from bottom to top, from the reality of medical processes towards abstraction and generalization, unlike the method generally specific to the philosophy of medicine which proceeds in the opposite direction, starting from a choice of premises of which it draws the consequences and seeks to apply to questions relating to medicine.

One of the originalities of this text is the thesis that medicine is not based on diseases, but on the logical priority of negativities: *Omnis determinatio est negativo* wrote Spinoza. It identifies what is abnormal and, within the limits of what is abnormal, decides what is pathological.

One of the first requirements of the philosophy of medicine is the need for clarification of a discipline that often uses terms that are imprecise, ambiguous and whose multiple meanings call for clarification. The philosophical literature has carried out and continues to carry out important and fruitful research on this subject.

It focuses on the concepts of physical and mental illness, health, causality, medical explanation, or diagnosis, but it avoids others, such as that of treatment, even though this is the primary motivation of the medical discipline.

L. Karhausen, *The Fragility of Philosophy of Medicine*, Philosophy and Medicine 147, https://doi.org/10.1007/978-3-031-41633-0_15

One of the difficulties comes from the fact that philosophers in their legitimate search for clarification seek, with intermittent success—and they are aware of this—to propose definitions based on necessary and sufficient criteria.

However, Wittgenstein has shown that this essentialist approach is misplaced and unnecessary. He suggests replacing this essentialist vision with that of a quorum of characteristics that he calls family resemblances. All concepts of medical language must then be re-examined in the light of this approach, which avoids endless debates on problems of definition and conceptual questions.

There is sometimes a certain distance between the philosophy of medicine and clinical medicine. It is necessary, but not always possible and rarely achieved, to translate the considerations of the first discipline into those of the second. Although they deal with problems that fall within the scope of medicine, the philosophers of medicine generally converse with each other. They address themselves to other philosophers but have few exchanges with those who practice clinical medicine or deal with public health. They sometimes develop philosophical speculations on a certain subject that conflict with relevant medical knowledge on the same subject.

Philosophy offers certainties but medicine constantly struggles against uncertainty.

References

1. ***Caplan AL.*** Does the Philosophy of Medicine Exist? *Theoretical Medicine.* 1992, **13 :** 67–77
2. ***Broadbent A.*** Philosophy of Medicine. Oxford University Press. 2019, xvii
3. ***Hull DL.*** Philosophy of Biological Science. Prentice Hall. 1974
4. ***Mahner M, Bunge M.*** Foundations of Biophilosophy. Springer. 1997
5. ***Marcum JA.*** (ed.). The Bloomsbury Companion to Contemporary Philosophy of Medicine. London. Bloomsbury. 2017. ***Solomon M.*** Making Medical Knowledge. Oxford University Press. 2015. ***Gifford F.*** Philosophy of Medicine. Handbook of Philosophy of Science. Volume 16. Amsterdam. Elsevier. 2011. ***Schramme T & S Edwards S.*** Handbook of the Philosophy of Medicine. Springer. 2017. ***Lee K.,*** The Philosophical Foundations of Modern Medicine. London. Palgrave MacMillan. 2012
6. ***Loughlin M, Bluhm R, Gupta M.*** Research Problems and Methods in the Philosophy of Medicine, in: ***JA Marcum,*** (ed.) The Bloomsbury Companion to Contemporary Philosophy of Medicine. Bloomsbury, 2017, pp. 56–57
7. ***Karhausen L.*** Les flux de la philosophie des sciences au 20e siècle. L'Harmattan. 2011
8. ***Karhausen L.*** Analytic Philosophy of Medicine. Reconsidering the Relation Between Philosophy of Science and Clinical Medicine. Austin Macauley Publishers. 2022
9. ***O'C Drury M.*** in: ***R. Rhees*** (ed.) Recollection of Wittgenstein. Oxford University Press. 1984, p.77
10. ***Tiercelin C.*** La métaphysique et les sciences. Les nouveaux enjeux. *Lato sensu. Revue de la société de philosophie des sciences.* **3: 1–16, 2016**
11. ***Grantham TA.*** Conceptualizing the (Dis)unity of Science. *Philosophy of Science.* **71:** 133–155, 2003
12. ***Dupré J.*** The Disorder of Things. Harvard University Press. 1993
13. ***Rosenberg A.*** instrumental Biology or the Disunity of Science. The University of Chicago Press. 1994, pp.20–22
14. ***Cartwright N.*** Nature's Capacities and their Measurement. Oxford. Clarendon Press. 1989. ***Cartwright N.*** The Dappled World: A Study of the Boundaries of Science. Cambridge University Press. 1999
15. ***Wittgenstein L.*** Philosophical Investigations. Blackwell. 1968 §§ 90, 97
16. ***Wittgenstein L.*** Philosophical Investigations. Blackwell.1968, II§174
17. ***Wittgenstein L.*** Zettel. Oxford. Basil Blackwell. 1967, §567
18. ***Wittgenstein L.*** Philosophical Remarks. Blackwell. 1975, §47
19. ***Wittgenstein L.*** On the philosophy of psychology. Vol. II. Blackwell. 1980, §727
20. ***Wittgenstein L.*** Remarks on the philosophy of psychology. Vol I Blackwell. 1980, §436

L. Karhausen, *The Fragility of Philosophy of Medicine*, Philosophy and Medicine 147, https://doi.org/10.1007/978-3-031-41633-0

21. ***Floyd J.*** Recent Themes in the History of Early Analytic Philosophy. *Journal of the History of Philosophy.* **47:** 157–200, 2009
22. ***Wittgenstein L.*** Private Notebooks 1914–1916. Norton & Company. 2022
23. ***Wittgenstein L.*** Philosophical Investigations. Blackwell. 1968., §569
24. ***Wittgenstein L.*** Philosophical Investigations. Blackwell. 1968, §§ 373, 371, §109
25. ***Wittgenstein L.*** Philosophical Investigations. Blackwell. 1968, §§ 373, 37. ***Ananth M.*** In defense of an evolutionary concept of health nature, norms, and human biology. Ashgate. Aldershot, 2008. ***Kovacs J.*** The concept of health and disease. *Medical Health Care Philosophy.* ***Wittgenstein L.*** Philosophical Investigations. Blackwell. 1968, §§ 373, 37
26. ***Soulez A.*** Wittgenstein et le tournant grammatical. Presses Unversitaires de France. 2004, p.32
27. ***Baker G.*** Wittgenstein's Depth Grammar in : Method. Neglected Aspects. Blackwell. 2006, pp.73–91
28. ***Wittgenstein L.*** Philosophical Investigations. Blackwell. 1968, §§32–35
29. ***Wittgenstein L.*** Philosophical Investigations. Blackwell. 1968, §497
30. ***Wittgenstein L.*** Zettel. Oxford. Basil Blackwell. 1967, 358
31. ***Wittgenstein L.*** Philosophical Investigations. Blackwell. 1968, §97
32. ***Wittgenstein L.*** Philosophical Investigations. Blackwell. 1968, §95
33. ***Wittgenstein L.*** Philosophical Remarks. Blackwell. 1975, p. 72
34. ***Wittgenstein L.*** Philosophical Investigations. Blackwell. 1968, §50
35. ***Wittgenstein L.*** Philosophical Investigations. Blackwell. 1968, §126
36. ***Plato.*** Le Grand Hippias, in: ***Plato.*** Œuvres complètes, I, Gallimard. Pléiade, 1950, pp. 22–56
37. ***Wittgenstein L.*** Philosophical Investigations. Blackwell. 1968, §§ 67, 77, 108, 164, 179, 236
38. ***Wittgenstein L.*** Philosophical Investigations. Blackwell. 1968, §67
39. ***Wittgenstein L.*** The Blue and Brown Book. Blackwell. 1968, p. 150
40. ***Wittgenstein L.*** Philosophical Investigations. Blackwell. 1968, §67
41. ***Wittgenstein L.*** Philosophical Investigations. Blackwell. 1968, §7
42. ***Wittgenstein L.*** Philosophical Investigations. Blackwell. 1968, §66
43. ***Wing L.*** The Autistic Spectrum. London. Constable. 1996, pp. 40–42
44. ***Wittgenstein L.*** Philosophical Investigations. Blackwell. 1968, §23
45. ***Wittgenstein L.*** Philosophical Investigations. Blackwell. 1968, §23
46. ***Ferrarese E, Laugier S.*** Formes de vie. Paris. CNRS. 2018
47. ***Wittgenstein L.*** Philosophical Investigations. Blackwell. 1968, §23
48. ***Rhees R.*** Discussions of Wittgenstein. Routledge and Kegan Paul. 1970, p. 278
49. ***Wittgenstein L.*** Philosophical Investigations. Blackwell. 1968, §23 & pp. 247–248. ***Wittgenstein L.*** Philosophical Investigations. Blackwell. 1968, §23 & pp. 247–248. ***Wittgenstein L.*** Philosophical Investigations. Blackwell. 1968, §23 & pp. 247–248
50. ***Wittgenstein*** L. Philosophische Untersuchungen. Blackwell.1968, IIxi, p. 223
51. ***Wittgenstein*** L. Philosophische Untersuchungen. Blackwell.1968, IIxi, p. 223
52. ***Wittgenstein L.*** Philosophical Investigations. Blackwell. 1968, §185–242
53. ***Wittgenstein*** L. Philosophical Investigations. Blackwell. 1968, §197–202. ***Wittgenstein L.*** Philosophical Grammar. Blackwell. 1974, pp.213–214
54. ***Wittgenstein L.*** Philosophical Remarks. Blackwell. 1975, §200–205
55. ***Wittgenstein L.*** Philosophical Investigations. Blackwell. 1968, §201–202, 217, 337
56. ***Wittgenstein L.*** Philosophical Investigations. Blackwell. 1968, §199
57. ***Kripke SA.*** Wittgenstein On Rules and Private Language. Blackwell. 1982
58. ***Wittgenstein L.*** Philosophical Investigations. Blackwell. 1968, §201
59. ***Margolis*** *J*. Negativities. The Limits of Life. Colombus. Ohio. Charles E. Merrill Publishing Company. 1975, p. 96
60. ***Margolis*** *J*. Negativities. The Limits of Life. Charles E. Merrill Publishing Company. 1975, 98–99
61. ***Downie RS***, Personal communication, 2007
62. ***Williams B.*** Ethics and the Limit of Philosophy. Harvard University Press. 1985
63. ***Nordin I.*** The Limits of Medical Practice. *Theoretical Medical Bioethics.* **20:** 105–123, 1999

64. ***Anscombe E***. Rules, Rights and Promises. Collected Papers. 1981, vol III: Chapter 10
65. ***Wittgenstein L.*** Philosophical Investigations. Blackwell. 1968, §383
66. ***Wittgenstein L.*** Philosophical Investigations. Blackwell. 1968, §116
67. ***Wittgenstein L.*** Philosophical Investigations. Blackwell. 1968, §43
68. ***Stewart M***. Patient-Centered Medicine. Transforming the Clinical Method. Thousand Oaks, California. Sage Publications. 1995; p. 33
69. ***Karhausen L.*** Mythologies médicales. L'Harmattan. 2014, pp. 149–163
70. ***Zakrison TL, Valdès DM, Muntaner C.*** Social Violence, Structural Violence, Hate, and the Trauma Surgeon. *International Journal of Health Services.* **49:** 665)681, 2019
71. ***Glover J***. What Sort of Persons should there be? London. Penguin Books. 1984. ***Harris J.*** Enhancing Evolution. The Ethical Case for Making Better People. Princeton University Press. 2007
72. ***James W.*** Pragmatism. Harvard University Press. 1907. 1979, 30
73. ***Illich I.*** Medical Nemesis. Penguin Books. 1978.
74. ***Aron D.*** Complex Systems in Medicine. Springer Link. 1979
75. ***Caplan et al.*** (eds.) Concepts of Health and Disease Interdisciplinary Perspectives. Addison-Wesley, 198, p. 41
76. ***Sedgwick P.*** Illness—mental and otherwise, in ***Caplan et al.*** (eds.) Concepts of Health and Disease Interdisciplinary Perspectives. Addison-Wesley, 1981, pp 119–129
77. ***Schopenhauer.*** The World as Will and Representation. New York. Dover. 1966, p. 180
78. ***Austin J.*** Quand lire c'est faire. Paris. Seuil. 1970, p. 80
79. ***Melamed YY.*** "Omnis detrminatio est negation": determination, negation, and self-negation in Spinoza, Kant, and Hegel. Chapter 10 in: ***F. Eckart n Y.Y. Melamed*** (eds.) Spinoza and German Idealism. Cambridge University Press. 2012, pp. 175–196
80. ***Broadbent A.*** Philosophy of Medicine. Oxford University Press. 2019, p. 125
81. ***Whitbeck C.*** Four Basic Concepts of Medical Science. *PSA* **1 :** 210–212, 1978
82. ***Wittgenstein L.*** Philosophical Investigations. Blackwell. 1968, §43
83. ***Cochrane AL.*** The history of the measurement of ill health. *International Journal of Epidemiology*. 1972 a **1** : 89
84. ***Rorty R.*** Inquiry as recontextualization: an anti-dualist account of interpretation, in: Objectivity, Relativism, and Truth, Philosophical Papers, vol. 1, Cambridge University Press, 1991
85. ***Banja JD.*** Defining Makes Perfect, in: ***JM Humber & RF Almeder*** (eds.) What is Disease? Towtowa, N.J. Humana Press, 1997, pp. 249–268
86. ***Wittgenstein L.*** The Blue and Brown Book. Blackwell. 1968
87. ***Wittgenstein L.*** The Blue and Brown Book. Blackwell. 1968
88. ***MacMahon B. & Trichpoulos D.*** Epidemiology Principles & Methods. Boston. Little Brown and Company. 1996
89. ***Osler W.*** Aequanimitas. P. Blakiston & Co. 1910
90. ***Wittgenstein L.*** Philosophical Investigations. Blackwell. 1968
91. ***Aron DC.*** Complex Systems in Medicine. Springer. 2020
92. ***Lycan W.*** Logical Form in Natural Language. Cambridge, Massachusetts. The MIT Press. 1985, 62–71
93. ***Jackson M.*** The Routledge History of Disease. Routledge. 2017
94. ***Payer L.*** Medicine and Culture. New York. Henry Holt and Company. 1988
95. ***Wolinsky H.*** Disease mongering and drug marketing. *EMBO Rep.* **6:** 612–614, 2005
96. ***De Bock C.*** L'industrie agro-alimentaire et la santé. *Éducation et Santé,* 311, Mai 2015
97. ***Wittgenstein L.*** The Blue and Brown Book. Blackwell. 1968
98. ***Simon J.*** Beyond naturalism and normativism. Reconceiving the « disease » debate. *Philosophical Papers.* **36:** 343–370, 2007
99. ***Sedgwick P.*** Illness — mental and otherwise. *Hastings Center Studies.* **1:** 19–40, 1973, pp. 30–31
100. ***Humber JM, Almeder RF.*** (eds.) What is a Disease? Humana Press. 1997
101. ***Wittgenstein L.*** The Blue and Brown Book. Blackwell. 1968

102. ***Caplan et al.*** (eds.) Concepts of Health and Disease Interdisciplinary Perspectives. Addison-Wesley, 198, p. 41
103. ***Sedgwick P.*** Illness—mental and otherwise, in ***Caplan et al.*** (eds.) Concepts of Health and Disease Interdisciplinary Perspectives. Addison-Wesley, 1981, pp 119–129
104. ***Wittgenstein L.*** Philosophical Investigations. Blackwell. 1968, §133
105. ***Wittgenstein L.*** Philosophical Investigations. Blackwell. 1968, §122
106. ***Ereshefsky M.*** Defining 'health' and 'disease'. *Studies in History and Philosophy of Science Part C: Studies in History and Philosophy of Biological and Biomedical Sciences.* **40:** 221–227, 2009
107. ***Platon.*** Phedra 265c–266b
108. ***Scadding JG.*** The clinician and the computer. *The Lancet.* **291:** 139–140, 1968
109. ***Bourse C.*** Health as a theoretical concept. *Philosophy of Science* **44:** 542–575, 1977
110. ***Hofmann B.*** Disease, illness and sickness, in ***M. Solomon, J.R. Simon, & H. Kincaid.*** The Routledge Companion to Philosophy of Medicine. London. Routledge, 2017, pp.16–26
111. ***Boorse C.*** On the distinction between disease and illness. *Philosophy & Public Affairs.* **5:** 49–68, 1975
112. ***Hare RM.*** Health. *Journal of Medical Ethics.* **12:** 174–181, 1986
113. ***Wakefield JC.*** The biostatistical theory versus the harmful dysfunction analysis, part 1 Is part-dysfunction a sufficient condition for medical disorder? *Journal of Medicine and Philosophy,* **39:** 648–682, 2014
114. ***Boorse C.*** A rebuttal on health, in: ***JM Humber & RF Almeder*** (eds.) What is Disease? Towtowa, N.J. Humana Press, 1997, pp. 3–134
115. ***Boorse C.*** A second rebuttal on health. *Journal of Medicine and Philosophy,* **39:** 683–724, 2014
116. ***Nordenfelt L.*** The concepts of health and illness revisited. *Medicine, Health Care and Philosophy,* **10:** 5–10, 2007
117. ***Clouter KD, Culver CM and Gert B.*** Malady, in: ***JM Humber & RF Almeder*** (eds.) What is Disease? Towtowa, N.J. Humana Press, pp. 175–217, 1977
118. ***Nesse RM & Stearns SC.*** The Great Opportunity: Evolutionary Applications to Medicine and Public Health. *Evolutionary Applications,* **1 :** 28–48, 1994
119. ***Méthot PO.*** À propos de la difficulté de définir la maladie : une perspective darwinienne, in : ***E. Giroux & M. Lemoine*** (eds.) Philosophie de la médecine. Santé, maladie, pathologie. Paris. Vrin. 2012, pp.177–213
120. ***Cournoyea M.*** Evolutionary Medicine, in: ***M. Solomon, J.R. Simon, & H. Kincaid.*** The Routledge Companion to Philosophy of Medicine. London. Routledge, 2017, pp. 475–486
121. ***Moore GE.*** Principia Ethica, §10 ¶ 3
122. ***Margolis J.*** The Concept of Disease. *The Journal of Medicine and Philosophy,* **1:** 238–255, 1976
123. ***Rezneck L.*** The nature of disease. Routledge and Kegan Paul. 1987
124. ***Cartwright SA.*** Report on the disease and physical peculiarities of the Negro race, in: ***A. Caplan, J. MacCartney & D. Sisti,*** (eds.) Health, Disease and Illness. Concepts in Medicine. Georgetown University Press. 2004, pp. 28–39
125. ***Spitzer RL.*** The diagnostic status of homosexuality: DSM-III. *American Journal of Psychiatry.* **138 :** 210–215, 1981
126. ***Foucault M.*** Histoire de la folie à l'âge Classique. Poche.1976
127. ***Szasz T.*** The Myth of Mental Illness. New York. Perennial. 1974
128. ***Conrad P.*** Discovery of hyperkinesis: Notes on the medicalization of deviant behavior. *Social Problems.* **23 :**12–21, 1975
129. ***Moynihan RN & Henry D.*** The fight against disease mongering: Generating knowledge for action. *PLoS Med.* 3, e191, 2006
130. ***Moynihan RN, Cooke GPE, Doust JA, et al.*** Expanding disease definitions in guidelines and expert panel ties to industry. A cross-sectional study of common conditions in the United States. *PLoS Med.* 10, e1001500, 2013

131. ***Conrad P.*** Discovery of hyperkinesis: Notes on the medicalization of deviant behavior. *Social Problems.* **23** :12–21, 1975
132. ***Batstra AL & Frances A.*** Diagnostic inflation: Causes and a suggested cure. *The Journal of Nervous and Mental Diseases.* **200:** 474–479, 2012
133. ***Chrisler JC & Gorman JA.*** The medicalization of women's moods; Premenstrual syndrome and premenstrual dysphoric disorder, in: The Wrong Prescription for Women: How Medicine and Media create a 'Need' for Treatments, Drugs and Surgery. Santa Barbara. Praeger Press, pp. 77–98, 2015
134. ***Carpiano RM.*** Passive medicalization. The case of Viagra and erectile dysfunction. *Sociological Spectrum.* **21:** 441–450, 2001
135. ***Strawson PF.*** Carnap's Views of Constructed Systems versus Natural Languages in analytic philosophy, in : ***Schilpp P.***(ed.) The Philosophy of Rudolf Carnap. Lasalle. Open Court. pp. 503–518
136. ***Searle J.*** La construction sociale de la réalité. Gallimard. 1998
137. ***Wittgenstein L.*** Philosophical Investigations. Blackwell. 1968, §124
138. ***Kingma E.*** Disease as Scientific and as Value-Laden Concept, in: ***T. & S. Edwards*** (eds.) Handbook of the Philosophy of Medicine. Springer. Vol. 1, 2017, pp. 45–63
139. ***Wakefield JC.*** The concept of mental disorder: On the boundary between biological facts and social values. *American Psychologist.* **47:** 373, 1992
140. ***Wakefield JC.*** The concept of mental disorder: Diagnostic implications of the harmful dysfunction analysis. *World Psychiatry.* **6:** 149–156, 2007
141. ***Wakefield JC.*** The biostatistical theory versus the harmful dysfunction analysis, part 1: Is part-dysfunction a sufficient condition for medical disorder. *Journal of Medicine and Philosophy.* **39:** 648–682, 2014
142. ***Engel GL.*** The biopsychological model and the education of health professionals. *Annals of the New York Academy of Sciences.* **310:** 169–181, 1978
143. ***Gifford F.*** The biomedical model and the biopsychosocial model on medicine, in: ***M. Solomon, J.R. Simon, & H. Kincaid.*** The Routledge Companion to Philosophy of Medicine. London. Routledge, 2017, pp. 445–454
144. ***Caplan AL.*** Is aging a disease? in: ***A.L. Caplan.*** *If I were a rich man could I buy a pancreas?* Bloomington. Indiana University Press., pp. 1295–209, 1992
145. ***Powell R, Scarffe E.*** "Rethinking Disease": a fresh diagnosis and a new philosophical treatment. *Journal of Medical Ethics.***45:** 579–588, 2019
146. ***Hacking I.*** Plasmare le persone. Corso al College de France (2004–2005)
147. ***Wittgenstein L.*** Philosophical Investigations. Blackwell. 1968, §17
148. ***Magd CS, Chiong W, Smith KC.*** Diagnosing and Defining Disease. Genetic Disease, Genetic Testing, and the Clinician. In the Twilight: Life in the Margins Between Sick and Well. *Journal of the American Medical Association.* **286:** 87–93, 2021
149. ***MacMahon B. & Trichpoulos*** Epidemiology Principles & Methods. Boston. Little Brown and Company. 1996, pp. 32–36
150. ***Wittgenstein L.*** The Blue and Brown Book. Blackwell. 1968, pp.19–20
151. ***Wittgenstein L.*** Philosophical Investigations. Blackwell. 1968, § 126
152. ***Margolis J.*** The Concept of Disease. *The Journal of Medicine and Philosophy,* **1** : 238–255, 1976, p.247
153. ***Rezneck L.*** The Nature of Disease. Routledge and Kegan Paul. 1987, 97
154. ***Steele A.*** Ageless. The New Science of Getting Older Without Getting Old. New York. Random House. 2020
155. ***Kerepesi C. et al.*** Epigenetic clocks reveal a rejuvenation event during embryogenesis followed by aging. *Science Advances*. Published online June 25, 2021. https://doi.org/10.1126/sciadv.abg6082.
156. ***Lehallier B, Gate D, Schaum N, Wyss-Coray T et al.*** Undulating changes in human plasma proteome profiles. *Nature Medicine.* **25** :1843–1850, 2019

157. ***Dong X, Milholland B, Vijg J.*** Evidence for a limit to human lifespan. *Nature* **538:** 257–259, 2016
158. ***Barbi E, Lagona F, Marsili M, Vaupel JW, Wachter KW.*** The Plateau of Human Mortality: Demography of Longenity Pioneers. *Science.* **360:** 1459–1461, 2019
159. ***Yuancheng L, Brommer B, Sinclair D.*** Reversal of biological clock restores vision in old mice. *Nature.* **588:** 124–129, 2020
160. ***Kinns H, Housley D, Freeman DB.*** Munchausen Syndrome and Factitious disorder: The Role of the Laboratory in the Detection and Diagnosis. *Annals of Clinical Biochemistry.* **50**: 194–203, 2013
161. ***Campbell EJM, Scadding JG, Roberts RS.*** The concept of disease. *British Medical Journal.* **2:** 757–762, 1979
162. ***Kendell RE.*** The Concept of Disease and its Implications for Psychiatry. *British Journal of Psychiatry.* **127:** 305–315, 1975
163. ***Stewart M, Tugwell P, MvWhinney L. et al.*** Patient-centered medicine: Transforming the Clinical Method. London. Radcliffe Publishing. 2014
164. ***McCarthy J., Rose P.*** Values-Based Health and Social Care.: Beyond Evidence Based Practice. London: Sage. 2010
165. ***Pickering N.*** Extending disorder: essentialism, family resemblance and secondary sense. *Medical Health Care and Philosophy.* **16:** 186–195, 2013
166. ***Bambrough R.*** Universals and Family Resemblances, in: ***G. Pitcher*** (ed.) Wittgenstein The Philosophical Investigations. New York. Anchor Books. 1961, pp. 186–204
167. ***Robins E, Guze SB.*** Establishment of Diagnostic Validity in Psychiatric Illness. Its Application to Schizophrenia. *American Journal of Psychiatry.* **126:** 983–987, 1970
168. ***Maj M, Gaebel W, López-lbor JJ, Sartorius N.*** Psychiatric Diagnosis and Classification. Wiley, 2002, pp. 14–15
169. ***Culver CM and Gert B***. Philosophy in Medicine. Conceptual and Ethical Issues in Medicine and Psychiatry. Oxford. Oxford University Press. 1982, 87–108. ***Nesse RM.*** Good Reasons for Bad Feelings. Penguin. Dutton. 2019, 128
170. ***Wing JK, Sartorius N, ÜstÜn TB.*** Diagnosis and clinical measurement in psychiatry. Cambridge. Cambridge University Press. 2017, 1
171. ***Van Nierop M, van Ios J ; Gunther M et al.*** Phenotypically continuous with clinical psychosis, discontinuous in need for care: evidence for an extended psychosis phenotype. *Schizophrenia Bulletin.* **38:** 231–238, 2012
172. ***Nuevo R, Chatterji S, Verdes E, et al.*** The continuous of psychotic symptoms in the general population: a cross-national study. *Schizophrenia Bulletin.* **38:** 475–485, 2012
173. ***Paris J.*** Is Psychoanalysis Still Relevant to Psychiatry? *Canadian Journal of Psychiatry.* **62**: 308–312, 2017
174. ***Hollingshead AB. and Redlich FC***. Social Class and Mental Illness. New York. 1958
175. ***Raballo A & Laroi F***. Clinical staging: a new scenario for the treatment of psychosis. *New England Journal of Medicine*. 2009; **374**: 365–367, 366
176. ***Skodol AE.*** Longitudinal course and outcome of personality disorders. *Psychiatric Clinics of North America.* 2008; **31**: 495–503
177. ***Nussbaum M.*** The Therapy of Desire. Theory and Practice in Hellenistic Ethics. Princeton. Princeton University Press. 1994, 51
178. ***Sims ACP.*** Symptoms in the Mind. Philadelphia. Saunders. 2003, 209–229
179. ***Glover J.*** I: The Philosophy and Psychology of Personal Identity. Penguin Books. 1988
180. ***Ramachandran VS.*** The Emerging Mind, lecture 2, Synapses of the Self. Reith Lectures: The Emerging Mind. BBC Radio 4, April 30, 2003
181. ***Laing RD.*** The Divided Self. London. Penguin Books. 1965
182. ***Jaynes J.*** The Origins of Consciousness in the Breakdown of the Bicameral Mind. London. Allen & Unwin. 1976
183. ***Sass LA.*** Les paradoxes dy délire. Ithaque. 2010, pp.122, 124–128

184. ***Sass LA.*** The Paradoxes of Delusion. Wittgenstein, Schreber, and the Schizophrenic Mind. Cornell University Press. 1994, p.88
185. ***Murphy D.*** Psychiatry in the Scientific Image. The MIT Press. 2006, pp. 232–235
186. ***Sass LA.*** The Paradoxes of Delusion. Wittgenstein, Schreber, and the Schizophrenic Mind. Cornell University Press. 1994, p.76–80
187. ***Rochester S & Martin J.*** Crazy Talk. A Study of the Discourse of Schizophrenic Speakers. New York. Plenum Press. 1979
188. ***Murphy D.*** Psychiatry in the Scientific Image. The MIT Press. 2006, pp. 231–235
189. ***Nagel E.*** Teleology Revisited and Other Essays in the Philosophy of Science. New York. Columbia University Press. 1979, 165
190. ***Nagel T.*** What is it like to be a bat? *Philosophical Review.* **83:** 435–450, 1974
191. ***Wittgenstein L.*** Philosophical Investigations. Blackwell. 1968, §123
192. ***Jaspers K.*** General Psychopathology. Manchester. Manchester University Press; 1962 p. 577
193. ***Putnam H.*** Reason, Truth and History. Cambridge. Cambridge University Press. 1981
194. ***Wittgenstein L.*** Philosophical Investigations. Blackwell. 1968, § 481
195. ***Bortolotti L.*** Rationality and sanity: the role of rationality judgments in understanding psychiatric disorders, 480–496, in: ***Fullford KWM, Davies M, Graham G.*** (eds.), 2013
196. ***Radden, J.*** Madness and Reason. London. Allen & Unwin. 1985, 43–71
197. ***Kant I.*** Versuch Über die Krankheiten des Kopfes, 259–271, in : Kant's Werke, Bd II–Gesammelte Schriften, Vorkritische Schr. II, 1757–1777, Berlin. Reimer. 1905
198. ***Murphy D.*** Psychiatry in the Scientific Image. The MIT Press. 2006, pp. 152–158, 198–199
199. ***Owen GS, Cutting J, Davis AS.*** Are people with schizophrenia more logical than healthy volunteers? *British Journal of Psychiatry.* **191:** 453–454, 2007
200. ***Margolis J.*** Psychotherapy & Morality. A study of two Concepts. New York. Random House. 1966, 11
201. ***Siegler M and Osmond H.*** Models of Madness, Models of Medicine. New York. MacMillan Publishing Co. 1974, 48
202. ***Nagel T.*** Mortal Questions. Cambridge. Cambridge University Press. 1979
203. ***Hacking I.*** The social construction of what? Cambridge. Harvard University Press. 1999, 104–105
204. ***Danto A.*** Analytical Philosophy of Knowledge. Cambridge. Cambridge University Press. 1968, 232
205. ***Arnold M.*** Culture and Anarchy: With Friendship's Garland and Some Literary Essays. Ann Arbor. University of Michigan Press. 1960, 167–168
206. ***Slavney PR, McHugh PR.*** Psychiatric Polarities. Methodology & Practice. The Johns Hopkins University Press. 1987, 71–84
207. ***Wyss D***, in: ***Havens LL.*** Approaches to the Mind. Boston. Little Brown and Company. 1973 359
208. ***Didi-Hubermann G.*** Invention de l'hystérie. Editions Macula. 2012
209. ***Sartorius N, Holt RIG, Maj M.*** Comorbidity of Mental Disorders and Physical Disorders. Basel. Karger. 2015
210. ***RittnerHL, Brack A, Stein C.*** Pro-algesic and analgesic actions of immune cells. *Current Opinions in Anaesthesiology.* **16 :** 527–533, 2003
211. ***Pitharouli MC, Hagenaars SP, Glanville KP, et al.*** Elevated C-Reactive Protein in Patients With Depression, Independent of Genetic, Health, and Psychosocial Factors: Results From the UK Biobank. *American Journal of Psychiatry.* May 14, 2021
212. ***Radavelli-Bagatini S, Naidoo U.*** *Clinical Nutrition.* Publié en ligne, 15 avril 1921
213. ***Kraepelin E.*** Lectures on Clinical Psychiatry. New York. William Wood and Company. 1913, 295
214. ***Hacking I.*** The social construction of what? Cambridge. Harvard University Press. 1999
215. ***Buckholz JW And Meyer-Lindenberg A.*** Psychopathology and the Human Connectome: Toward a Transdiagnostic Model of Risk for Mental Illness. *Neuron.***74:** 990–1004, 2012

216. ***Sartorius N, Holt RIG, Maj M.*** Comorbidity of Mental Disorders and Physical Disorders. Basel. Karger. 2015
217. ***Tinetti ME.*** Potential pitfalls of disease-specific guidelines for patients with multiple conditions. *New England Journal of Medicine.* 2004; **351:** 2870–2874, 2870
218. ***Lewis. A.*** Prognosis in the manic-depressive psychosis. *Lancet.* 1936; **55**: 997–999
219. ***Robins LN, Helzer JE, et al.*** Lifetime prevalence of specific psychiatric disorders in three sites. *Archives of General Psychiatry.* 1984; 949–958
220. ***Straus JS.*** Hallucinations and delusions as points on continuous function: rating scale evidence. *Archives of General Psychiatry.* **21:** 581–586, 1969
221. ***Van Fraassen BC.*** The Scientific Image. Oxford University Press. 1980
222. ***Kendell RE and Jablensky A.*** Distinguishing between the validity and utility of psychiatric diagnoses. *American Journal of Psychiatry.* **160:** 4–12, 2003
223. ***Jablensky A.*** Psychiatric Classifications: validity and utility. *World Psychiatry.* **15:** 26–31, 2016
224. ***Campaner R.*** Varieties of Causal Explanation in Medical Contexts. Mimesis International. 2019
225. ***Jablensky A.*** A commentary on 'A proposal for a meta)-structure for DSM-5 and ICD-11. *Psychological Medicine.* 2009; **39:** 2099–2103, 2099
226. ***Marks EM., Hunter MS.*** Medically Unexplained Symptoms: an acceptable term? *British Journal of Pain* 2015; **9**: 109–114
227. ***Klaus K., Rief W., Brähler E. et al.*** The distinction between "medically unexplained" and "medically explained" in the context of somatoform disorders. *International Journal of Behavioral Medicine.* 2013; **20** :161–71
228. ***Jablensky A and Kendell RE.*** Criteria for assessing a classification in psychiatry, 1–24, in: ***Maj M., Gaebel W., Lopez-Ibor JJ. and Sartorius N.*** (eds.). Psychiatric Diagnosis and Classification. Chichester. Wiley & Sons. 2002, 22
229. ***Sartorius N.*** Mon combat pour la santé mentale. Odile Jacob. 2010
230. ***Rosenhan SL.*** On Being Sane in Insane Places. *Science***.** **179:** 250–258, 1973
231. ***Seligman MEP, Walker EF, Rosenhan DL.*** Psychopatologia. Selig ed. Poznań : Zysk i S-ka Publishing House ; 2003. p.268–323
232. ***Waismann F.*** Verifiability, in: Logic and Language, 1st series, **A Flew** (ed.), Oxford. Oxford University Press. 1953, 120
233. ***Strawson PF.*** Individuals. An Essay in Descriptive Metaphysics. London. Methuen. 1959, 110
234. ***Barraclough B. et al.*** A Hundred Cases of Suicides: Clinical Aspects. *British Journal of Psychiatry.* 1974; 355–373
235. ***Putnam H.*** Mind Language and Reality. Philosophical papers. Volume 2. Cambridge. Cambridge University Press. 1975, 429–440
236. ***Gandal MJ, Haney JR, Parikshak NN, Leppa V et al.*** Shared molecular neuropathology across major psychiatric disorders parallels polygenic overlap. *Science.* 2018; **359**: 693–697
237. ***Davidson D.*** Mental events, in: Actions and Events. Oxford. Clarendon Press. 1980
238. ***Kandel E.*** Psychiatry, Psychoanalysis and the New Biology of Mind. Arlington. American Scientific Publishing. 2005, Ch. 2
239. ***Murphy D.*** Psychiatry in the Scientific Image. The MIT Press. 2006, pp. 115–120
240. ***Fulford KWM, Thornton T, Graham G.*** Oxford Textbook of Philosophy of Psychiatry. Oxford University Press. 2006
241. ***Olbert CM, Gala GJ.*** Supervenience and Psychiatry. Are mental disorders brain disorders? *Journal of Theoretical and Philosophical Psychology.* **35 :** 203–219, 2015
242. ***Jamison KR***. De l'exaltation à la dépression : confession d'une psychiatre maniaco-dépressive, Robert Laffont. 1997
243. ***Sandison RA.*** Depression: illness, social disease, or natural state? *Lancet.*1972; **299**: 1227–1229., 1228

244. ***Tas J***. Psychical disorders among inmates of concentration camps and repatriates. *Psychiatric Quarterly*. 1951; **25**: 683–685
245. ***Alloy LB. and Abramson LY***. Depressive realism: four theoretical perspectives, in: **Alloy LB,** (ed.) Cognitive Processes in Depression. New York. Guilford. 1988
246. ***Laing RD.*** The Divided Self. London. Penguin Books. 1965, 195
247. ***Nesse RM.*** Good Reasons for Bad Feelings. Penguin. Dutton. 2019, 89–94
248. ***WHO.*** Report of the International Pilot Study of Schizophrenia. World Health Organisation 1973
249. ***Haukka J, Suvisaari J, Lonnqvist J.*** Fertility of patients with schizophrenia, their siblings, and the general population: a cohort study from 1950 to 1959 in Finland. *American Journal of Psychiatry.* **160:** 460–463, 2007
250. ***Jablensky A.*** The diagnostic concept of schizophrenia: its evolution, and future prospects. *Dialogues in Clinical Neuroscience.* **12:** 271–287, 2010
251. ***Keller MC, Miller G.*** Resolving the paradox of common, harmful, heritable mental disorders: which evolutionary genetic models work best? *Behavioural Brain Science.* **29:** 385–404, 2006
252. ***Perarlson GD, Folley BS.*** Schizophrenia, Psychiatric Genetics, and Darwinian Psychiatry: An Evolutionary Framework. *Schizophrenia Bulletin.* **34:** 722–733, 2008
253. ***Silverman J.*** Shamans and Acute Schizophrenia. *American Anthropologist.* 1967; **69**: 21–31
254. ***Benedict R.*** Patterns of Culture. Boston. 1934
255. ***Jaynes J.*** The Origin of Consciousness in the Breakdown of the Bicameral World. Houghton Mifflin. Boston. 1976
256. ***McGilchrist I.*** the Master and His Emissary. The Divided Brain and the Making of the Western World. Yale University Press. 2019
257. ***Fulford KWM, Thornton T, Graham G.*** Oxford Textbook of Philosophy of Psychiatry. Oxford University Press. 2006
258. ***Sass LA.*** Incomprehensibility and Understanding: On the Interpretation of Severe Mental Illness. *Philosophy, Psychiatry, & Psychology.* **10:** 125–132n 2020
259. ***Wittgenstein L.*** Philosophical Investigations. Blackwell. 1968, §122
260. ***Fuchs T.*** Delusion, Reality and Intersubjectivity. *Philosophy, Psychiatry and Psychology,* **27:** 61–79, 2020
261. ***Sass LA.*** Contradictions of Emotions in Schizophrenia. *Cognition & Emotion.* **21:** 351–390, 2007
262. ***Wittgenstein L.*** Culture and Values. Oxford. Blackwell. 1980
263. ***Sechehaye M,*** (ed.) Autobiography of a schizophrenic girl. New American Library. 1970, p. 33
264. ***Sass LA.*** The Paradoxes of Delusion. Wittgenstein, Schreber, and the Schizophrenic Mind. Cornell University Press. 1994, p.8
265. ***Sass LA.*** The Paradoxes of Delusion. Wittgenstein, Schreber, and the Schizophrenic Mind. Cornell University Press. 1994, p. 117
266. ***Read R.*** On approaching schizophrenia through Wittgenstein. *Philosophical Psychology.* **14:** 449–475, 2001
267. ***Read R.*** Wittgenstein among the Sciences. Routledge. 2012, p. 138
268. ***Read R.*** On Delusions of Sense: A Response to Coetzee and Sass. *Philosophy, Psychology and Psychiatry.* **10 :** 135–141, 2003
269. ***Schopenhauer A.*** Le monde comme volonté et représentation. Gallimard. 2009 ? pp. 251–252
270. ***Wittgenstein L.*** Philosophical Investigations. Blackwell. 1968, §410
271. ***Wittgenstein L.*** Philosophical Investigations. Blackwell. 1968, §398
272. ***Aucouturier V, Demazeux S.*** The Concept of "Mental Disorder", in: ***H. Carel, Cooper R.*** (eds.) Health, Illness and Disease. Routledge. 2013, p. 83
273. ***Lilienfeld SO, Marino L.*** Mental Disorder as a Roschian Concept: A Critique of Wakefield's "Harmful Dysfunction" Analysis. *Journal of Abnormal Psychology.* **104:** 411–420, 1995

274. ***Lalumera E.*** Understanding Schizophrenia Through Wittgenstein: Empathy, Explanation and Philosophical Clarification, in: ***Hippolito I, Gonçalves J, Pereira J*** (eds.) Schizophrenia and Common Sense. Springer Nature. 2017
275. ***Van Duppen Z, Sips R.*** Understanding the Blind Spots of Psychosis: A Wittgensteinian and First-Person Approach. *Psychopathology.* **51:** 276–284, 2018
276. ***Wittgenstein L.*** On certainty. Blackwell.1969, §225
277. ***Wittgenstein L.*** The Blue and Brown Book. Blackwell. 1968
278. ***Van Duppen Z, Sips R.*** Understanding the Blind Spots of Psychosis: A Wittgensteinian and First-Person Approach. *Psychopathology.* **51:** 276–284, 2018, p. 283
279. ***Zola IK.*** Culture and symptoms—An analysis of patients' presenting complaints. *American Sociological Review.* 1966 ; 31 : 615–630 ; 617
280. ***Lemoine M.*** Introduction à la philosophie des sciences médicales. Paris. Hermann. 2017, p.6
281. ***Shorter E.*** From Paralysis to fatigue. A History of Psychosomatic Illnesses in the Modern Era. New York. The Free Press. 1992, 213
282. ***Weiner H and Fawzy IF.*** An Integrative Model of Health, Disease and Illness, 9–44, in: **Cheren, S** (ed.). Psychosomatic Medicine: Theory, Physiology and Practice, vol I. Madison, Conn. International Universities Press. 1989
283. ***Marks EM, Hunter MS.*** Medically Unexplained Symptoms: an acceptable term? *British Journal of Pain* 2015; **9**: 109–114
284. ***Klaus K, Rief W, Brähler E et al.*** The Distinction Between « Medically Unexplained » and « Medically Explained » Disorders in the Context of Somatoform Disorders. *International Journal of Behavioral Medicine.* **20:** 161–171, 2013
285. ***Dunnell K and Cartwright A.*** Medicine Takers, Prescribers and Hoarders. London. Routledge and Kegan Paul. 1972, 13
286. ***Verbrugge LM. & Ascione FJ.*** Exploring and iceberg. Common symptoms and how people care for them. *Medical Care.* 1987; **25**: 539–563
287. ***Wadsworth M, Butterfield W and Blaney R.*** Health and Sickness: The Choice of Treatment. London. Tavistock. 1979
288. ***Comaroff J***, in: **Shorter E.** Bedside Manners: The Troubled History of Doctors and Patients. New York. Simon & Schuster. 1985 p. 216
289. ***Cartwright A.*** Patients and Their Doctors: A Study of General Practice. London. Routledge. 1967
290. ***Stewart M., Brown JB., Weston WW. et al.*** Patient-Centered Medicine. Transforming the Clinical Method. Thousand Oaks, California. Sage Publications. 1995,33
291. ***Reidenberg MM and Lowenthal DT.*** Adverse non-drug reactions. *New England Journal of Medicine.* 1968; **279**: 678–679
292. ***Steinbrecher*** Causality. Philosophical Theory Meets Scientific Practice. Oxford University Press. 2014*N, **Koerber S, Frieser D and Hiller W.*** The Prevalence of Medically Unexplained Symptoms in Primary Care. *Psychosomatics.* 2011; **52:** 263–271
293. ***Simon GE., Gater R., Kisely S & Piccinelli M.*** Somatic symptoms of distress: an international primary care survey. *Psychosomatic Medicine.* 1996; **58**: 481–488
294. ***Alexander F.*** Psychosomatic Medicine. New York. Norton. 1950
295. ***Angell M.*** Disease as a reflection of the psyche. *The New England Journal of Medicine.* 1985a ; **312** : 1570–1572
296. ***Aronowitz RA.*** When do symptoms become a disease? *Annals of Internal Medicine.* 2001; **134**: 803–808
297. ***Bensing JM and Verhaak PFM.*** Somatization: a joint responsibility of doctor and patient. *New England Journal of Medicine.* 2006 **367**: 452–453
298. ***Zuger A.*** Dissatisfaction with medical practice. *New England Journal of Medicine.* 2004; **350**: 69–75
299. ***Hacking I.*** The social construction of what? Cambridge. Harvard University Press. 1999, 10
300. ***Rippere V.*** 'Hysteria", 'functional' or 'psychogenic'. *Journal of the Royal Society of Medicine.* 1992 ; **85** : 59–60

301. ***Karhausen L.*** Quand ls médias propagent des maladies fictives, in : ***L. Karhausen.*** Mythologies médicales. L'Harmattan. 2014, pp.149–163
302. ***Trimble MR.*** Functional diseases. *British Medical Journal.* 1982; **285**: 1768–1770, p.1768
303. ***Simon GE., Gater R., Kisely S & Piccinelli M.*** Somatic symptoms of distress: an international primary care survey. *Psychosomatic Medicine.* 1996; **58**: 481–488
304. ***Kirmayer LJ, Robbins JM.*** Three forms of somatization in primary care. Prevalence, co-occurrence, and sociodemographic characteristics. *The Journal of Nervous and Mental Disease.* 1991; **179**: 647–655. ***Simon GE., Von Korff M., Piccinelli M., Fullerton C. and Ormel J.*** An international study of the relation between somatic symptoms and depression. *The New England Journal of medicine.* 1999; **341**: 1329–1335. ***Barsky AJ.*** The patient with hypochondriasis. *The New England Journal of medicine.* 2001b **345** :1395–1399. ***Aaron LA and Buchwald D.*** A review of the evidence for overlap among unexplained clinical conditions. *Annals of Internal Medicine.* 2001 ; **134** : 868–880
305. ***Prins JB, van der Meer JW & Bleijenberg G.*** Chronic fatigue syndrome. *New England Journal of Medicine.* 2006; **467**: 346–355
306. ***Callahan D.*** The WHO definition of health. *Studies of the Hastings Center.* **1:** 77–87, 1973
307. ***Wylie C.*** The definition and measurement of health and disease. *Public Health Report.* **85:** 100–104, 1970
308. ***Kass LR.*** Regarding the End of Medicine and the Pursuit of Health. *Public Interest,* **40:** 11–42, 1975
309. ***Jadad AR, O'Grady L.*** How should health be defined? *BMJ.* 337: a2900. 2008
310. ***Boorse C.*** Health as a theoretical concept. *Philosophy of Science.* **44:** 542–573, 1977
311. ***Caplan A.*** The concept of health, illness, and disease, ***in***: ***W. Bynum & R. Porter*** (eds) Companion encyclopedia of the history of medicine, vol I, Routledge, 1993, pp. 233–248
312. ***Beauchamp T. and Childless J.*** Principles of biomedical ethics. 5th edition. Oxford University Press. 2001
313. ***Dupré J.*** Natural kinds and biological taxa. *The Philosophical Review.* **XC:** 66–91, 1981
314. ***Sholl J & Rattan SIS.*** Explaining Health Across the Sciences. Springer. 202
315. ***Kovacs J.*** The concept of health and disease. *Medical Health Care Philosophy.* **1:** 33–48, 1998
316. ***Ananth M.*** In defense of an evolutionary concept of health nature, norms, and human biology. Ashgate. Aldershot, 2008
317. ***Nordenfelt L.*** On the nature of health. An action-theoretic approach. Dordrecht. Reidel Publishing Company. 1987
318. ***Nordenfelt L.*** Quality of life, health and happiness. Averbury, Aldershot, 1993
319. ***Ereshefsky M.*** Defining 'health' and 'disease'. *Studies in History and Philosophy of Biological and Biomedical Sciences.* **40**: 221–227, 2009
320. ***Schramme T.*** A qualified defense of a naturalist theory of health. *Medicine, Health Care and Philosophy.* **10:** 11–17, 2007j
321. ***Varga S.*** Defining mental disorder. Exploring the 'natural function' approach. *Philosophy Ethics and Humanities in Medicine.* **6:** 1, 2017
322. ***Huber M, Knottnerus J, Green L et al.*** How should we define health? *British Medical Journal* 343: d4163
323. ***Hare RM.*** Health. *Journal of Medical Ethics.* **12:** 174–181, 1981
324. ***Brüssow H.*** What is health? *Microbial Biotechnology.* **6**: 341–348, 2013, pp.343–344
325. ***Schroeder SA.*** Rethinking Health: Healthy or Healthier Than? *The British Journal for the Philosophy f Science.* **64:** 131–159, 2013
326. ***Wittgenstein L.*** Vermischte Bemerkungen. Blackwell. 1978
327. ***Bognar G. & Hirose I.*** The Ethics of Health Care Rationing. An Introduction. London. Routledge, 2014, p.30
328. ***Broome J.*** Measuring the Burden of Disease by Aggregating Well-Being, in: ***C. Murray, S. Salomon, C. Mathers & A. Lopez*** (eds) Summary Measures of Population Health Concepts, Ethics, Measurement and Appplication. Geneva. World Health Organization, 2002, p. 94

329. ***Vanderweele T, Chen Y, Long K et al.*** Positive Epidemiology? *Epidemiology.* **31:** 189–193, 2020. ***Vanderweele T, McNeely E, Koh HK.*** Reimagining Health-Flourishing. *Journal of the American Medical Association.* **321:** 1667–1668, 2019
330. ***Aucouturier V, Demazeux S.*** The Concept of "Mental Disorder", in : ***H. Carel, Cooper R.*** (eds.) Health, Illness and Disease. Routledge. 2013, p. 78
331. ***MacMahon B. & Trichpoulos D.*** Epidemiology Principles & Methods. Boston. Little Brown and Company. 1996, p.19
332. ***Karhausen L.*** Causation: The elusive grail of epidemiology. *Medicine, Health Care and Philosophy.* **3:** 59–§è, 2000
333. ***MacMahon B. & Trichpoulos*** Epidemiology Principles & Methods. Boston. Little Brown and Company. 1996, pp.19–29
334. ***Giroux E.*** Contribution à l'histoire de l'épidémiologie des facteurs de risque. *Revue d'histoire des sciences.* **64:** 224, 2011. ***Broadbent A.*** Philosophy of Epidemiology, in ***J.A. Marcom,*** (ed.) The Bloomsbury Companion to anifestatContemporary Philosophy of Medicine. London. Bloomsbury, 2017
335. ***MacMahon B. & Trichpoulos D.*** Epidemiology Principles & Methods. Boston. Little Brown and Company. 1996, p.1 & 16
336. ***Karhausen L.*** Causation. The elusive grail of epidemiology. *Medicine, Health Care and Philosophy.* **3:** 59–67, 2000
337. ***Cartwright N.*** Hunting Causes and Using them. Cambridge University Press. 2007
338. ***Aristote.*** Metaphysics. Livre IX, chapter V
339. ***Hume D.*** Treatise of Human Nature. I, III, 14
340. ***Wittgenstein L.*** Philosophical Occasions 1912–1951, Cause and Effect. Hackett Publishing Company. 1993, p. 407
341. ***Mackie KL.*** *The Cement of the Universe. A Study of Causation.* Oxford: The Clarendon Press. 1974
342. ***Rothmann KJ.*** Causes. *American Journal of Epidemiology.* **104:** 587–592, 1976
343. ***MacMahon B. & Trichpoulos D.*** Epidemiology Principles & Methods. Boston. Little Brown and Company. 1996
344. ***Wittgenstein L.*** *Tractatus logico-philosophicus.* Routledge & Kegan Paul. 1922, §6.33–6.341, §6.36f, §6.362
345. ***Wittgenstein L.*** *Tractatus logico-philosophicus.* Routledge & Kegan Paul. 1922. § 6.32
346. ***Wittgenstein L.*** Wittgenstein's Lectures. Cambridge 1932–1935. Blackwell. 1982, p.16
347. ***Wittgenstein L.*** Philosophical Investigations. Blackwell. 1968, XII. ***Wittgenstein L.*** On Certainty. Blackwell. 1969, §368
348. ***Wittgenstein L.*** Cause and Effect. Intuitive Awareness., in: ***R. Rhees*** (ed.) *Philosophia.* 392–475, §24.9, 1976
349. ***Di Paola M.*** The Scapegoat Theory of Causality. The Creative Commons General Public License « Attribution, Non-Commercial; Share-Amoke », version 3.0 (CCPL BY-NC-SA), 2013
350. ***Wittgenstein L.*** Philosophical Investigations. Blackwell. 1968, §220
351. ***Wittgenstein L.*** Zettel. Oxford. Basil Blackwell. 1967, §296
352. ***Wittgenstein L.*** Philosophical Investigations. Blackwell. 1968, §169
353. ***Wittgenstein L.*** Philosophical Investigations. Blackwell. 1968, §§109, 126, 496
354. ***Wittgenstein L.*** Remarks on the Foundations of Mathematics. Blackwell, 1967, 333
355. ***Karhausen L.*** Causation in Epidemiology: a Socratic Dialogue: Plato. *International Journal of Epidemiology.* **30:** 704–706, 2001
356. ***von Wright GH.*** Explanation and Understanding. Ithaca. Cornell University Press. 1971
357. ***Shaffner K.*** Discovery and Explanation in Biology and Medicine. University of Chicago Press. 1993. Pp. 307–312
358. ***Kincaid H.*** Causal modelling mechanisms, and probability in epidemiology, in: ***I.P. Illari, F. Russo, J.*** **Williamson** (eds.) Causality in the Sciences. Oxford University Press. 2011, pp. 70–90

359. ***Reis J.*** Causality and Causal Inference in Medicine, in: ***M. Solomon, JR. Simon, H. Kincaid.*** (Eds.) The Routledge Companion to Philosophy of Medicine. London. Routledge, 2017, pp. 65–67
360. ***Hume D.*** An Enquiry Concerning Human Understanding. Clarendon Press. 1902, section VII, part II
361. ***Morgan SL, Winship C.*** Counterfactuals and Causal Inference. Cambridge University Press. 2007
362. ***Lewis DK.*** Counterfactuals. Blackwell. 1973
363. ***MacMahon B & Trichopoulos D.*** Epidemiology Principles and Methods. Boston. Little Brown and Company 1996, pp. 26–27
364. ***Vandenbroucke JP, Broadbent A, Pearce N.*** Causality and causal inference in epidemiology: the need for a pluralistic approach. *International Journal of Epidemiology.* **45:**1776–1786, 2016
365. ***Illary P, Russo F.*** Causality. Philosophical Theory Meets Scientific Practice. Oxford University Press. 2014
366. ***Jureidini J, McHenry LB.*** The Illusion of Evidence-Based Medicine. Exposing the crisis of credibility in clinical research. Wakefield Press. 2020
367. ***Putnam H.*** Naturalism, Realism and Normativity. Harvard University Press. 2016, p. 71
368. ***Cartwright N.*** Hunting Causes and Using Them. Cambridge University Press. 2007b
369. ***Danto A.*** Connections to the World. The Basic Concepts of Philosophy. New York. Harper & Row, Publishers. 1989, p. 258
370. ***Tallis R.*** Freedom: An Impossible Reality. Agenda Publishing. 2021, p. 79
371. ***Cartwright N.*** Nature's Capacities and their Measurement. Oxford. Oxford University Press. 1989
372. ***Skyrms B.*** Conditional Chance,161–178, in; ***Fetzer JH.*** (ed.). Probability and Causality. Dordrecht. Reidel Publishing Company. 1988. Pp. 172–176
373. ***Pearl J.*** Causality. Models, Reasoning, and Inference. Cambridge. Cambridge University Press. 2009. ***Pearl J.*** An Introduction to Causal Inference. *International Journal of Biostatistics.* 2010; **6**: Issue 2. Article 7
374. ***Pearl J, Glymour M, Jewell NP.*** Causal Inference in Statistics. Wiley. 2016
375. ***Cartwright N.*** Nature, the Artful Modeler. Open Court. Chicago. 2019, p. 82
376. ***McGrath J, Saha S, et al.*** Schizophrenia: a concise overview of medicine, prevalence, and mortality. *Epidemiological Review,* **30:** 67–76, 2008
377. ***MacMahon B. & Trichpoulos D.*** Epidemiology Principles & Methods. Boston. Little Brown and Company. 1996
378. ***Beckner M.*** The biological way of thought. Columbia University Press, New York, (1959).
379. ***Kripke S.*** Naming and Necessity. Harvard University Press. 1989
380. ***Wittgenstein L.*** The Blue and Brown Book. Blackwell. 1968
381. ***Wittgenstein L.*** Philosophical Investigations. Blackwell. 1968, §354
382. ***Fitelson B, Hitchcock C.*** Probabilistic measures of causal strength, in: ***P.M. Illari, F. Russo, J. Williamson*** (eds.) Causality in the Sciences. Oxford University Press. 2011, pp.601–627
383. ***Von Wright GH.*** Wittgenstein on Probability, pp. 139–162, in: ***G.H. von Wright,*** Wittgenstein. Blackwell. 1982
384. ***Sniderman AD, Navar AM, Thanassoulis G.*** Apolipoprotein B vs Low-Density Lipoprotein Cholesterol and Non-High Density Lipoprotein Cholesterol as the Primary Measure of Apolipoprotein B Lipoprotein-Related Risk. *JAMA Cardiology.* **7:** 257–258, 2022. ***Liu C, Dhindsa D, Almuwaqqat Z, Mehta A, Alkhoder AA et al.*** Association Between High-Density Lipoprotein Cholesterol Levels and Adverse Cardiovascular Outcomes in High-risk Populations. JAMA Cardiology. 7: 672–680, 2022
385. ***Giroux E.*** Le risque de maladie : normal ou pathologique ? in : Science, Philosophie et Société. Presses Universitaires de Franche-Comté. 2021, pp. 103–116
386. ***Holland W, Olsen JK & Du V. Florey.*** The Development of Modern Epidemiology: Personal Reports From Those Who Were There. Oxford University Press. 2007, p. 211

387. ***Susser M, Stein Z.*** Eras in Epidemiology. The Evolution of Ideas. Oxford University Press. 2009, pp.330–332
388. ***Lash TL, VanderWeele TJ, Haneuse S, Rothman KJ.*** Modern Epidemiology. Wolters Kluwer. 2021
389. ***Bhopal RS.*** Concepts of Epidemiology. Oxford University Press. 2016. p.33
390. ***Aschengrau A, Seage III GR.*** Essentials of Epidemiology. Jones and Bartlett Learning. 2020, p. 398–399
391. ***MacMahon B & Trichopoulos D.*** Epidemiology Principles and Methods. Boston. Little Brown and Company 1996, pp. 46–50.
392. ***Pelters B.*** Doing health, in: ***R. Cooper, H. Carels*** (eds.) Health, Illness and Disease. Durham: Acumen. 2013, pp. 197–210
393. ***Skrabanek P, & McCormick J.*** Follies & Fallacies in Medicine. New York. Prometheus Books. 1990, pp. 43–44
394. ***WHO*** collaborative study of neoplasia and steroid contraceptives: Invasive cervical cancer and combined oral contraceptive. *British Medical Journal.* **290:** 961–963, 1985
395. ***Fortney JA, Potts M, Bonhommre M.*** Invasive cancer and oral contraceptives. *British Medical Journal.* **290:** 1587–1589, 1985
396. ***Bhopal RS.*** Concepts of Epidemiology. Oxford University Press. 2016, pp. 221–223
397. ***Aronowitz RA.*** The converged experience of risk and disease. *Milbank Quarterly.* **87:** 417–442,
398. ***Karlawish J.*** How are we going to live with Alzheimer's disease? *Health Affairs.* **33:** 541–546, 2014
399. ***Howard J.*** Cognitive Errors and Diagnostic Mistakes. Springer. 2019, p.160
400. ***Maher B.*** The search for genome 'dark matter' moves closer. *Nature*. November 17, 2008. ***Visscher PM, Brown MA, McCarthy MI, Yang J.*** Five years of GWAS discovery. *American Journal of Human Genetics.* **90:** 7–24, 2012
401. ***Gejman PV, Sanders AR and Duan J.*** The Role of Genetics in the Etiology of Schizophrenia. *Psychiatric Clinics of North America.* **33:** 35–66, 2010
402. ***Illari P, Russo F, Williamson J.*** (Eds.) Causality in the Sciences. Oxford University Press. 2011. ***Illari P, Russo F.*** Causality. Philosophical Theory Meets Scientific Practice. Oxford University Press. 2014
403. ***Coste J***. Causal and Probabilistic Inference in Diagnostic Reasoning. & Giroux E. Risk Factors and Causality in Epidemiology, in: ***Huhneman P, Lambert G, Siberstein M.*** (eds.) Classification, Disease and Evidence. Springer. 2015
404. ***Wittgenstein L.*** Philosophical Investigations. Blackwell 1968, §109
405. ***Lovelock J***. Novacene. London. Allen Lane. 2019, p. 18
406. ***Thagard P.*** How Scientists Explain Diseases. Princeton. Princeton University Press. 1999, pp. 40–70
407. ***Davidson D.*** Causal relations. *Journal of Philosophy.* 1967; **64:** 691–703
408. ***Anscombe, G E M.*** "Causality and Extensionality." *The Journal of Philosophy.* **6**: 152–159. 1969
409. ***Skrabanek, Petr***. The Emptiness of the Black Box. *Epidemiology* **5.** 553–555. 1994
410. ***Strawson PF.*** "Causation and explanation", 115–135, in: ***B Vermazen, and M Hintikka*** (eds.). Essays on ***Davidson D.*** Actions and Events. Oxford. Clarendon Press. 1985, 126
411. ***Cunningham TV.*** Objectivity, Scientificity, and the Dualist Epistemology of Medicine, in: ***Huhneman P, Lambert G, Siberstein M.*** (eds.) Classification, Disease and Evidence. Springer. 2015
412. ***Harman G.*** The Inference to the Best Explanation. *Philosophical Review.* **74:** 88–95. 1965
413. ***Lash T, Vanderveele TJ, Haneuse s, Rothman J.*** Modern Epidemiology. Wolters Kluwer. 2021, pp. 7–9
414. ***Parascandola M.*** Epistemic risk: empirical evidence and the fear of being wrong. *Probability and Risk.* 2010: **9:** 201–214

415. ***Solomon M, Simon JR, Kincaid H.*** The Routledge Companion to Philosophy of Medicine. London. Routledge, 2017, pp. 385–389
416. ***Pearl J.*** Causality: Models, Reasoning and Inference. Cambridge University Press.2009. ***Nardini C.*** Bayesian versus frequentist clinical trials, in: ***M. Solomon, JR. Simon, H. Kincaid.*** The Routledge Companion to Philosophy of Medicine. London. Routledge, 2017, pp. 229–236
417. ***Thompson RP, Upshur EG.*** Philosophy of Medicine. An Introduction. Routledge. 2018, pp. 102–104
418. ***Cartwright N.*** What is Wrong with Bayes Nets? *The Monist.* **84 :** 242–264, 2001
419. ***Wittgenstein L.*** Philosophical Investigations. Blackwell. 1968, § 132
420. ***Anscombe E.*** Causality and Determinism, in: Metaphysics and The Philosophy of Mind. University of Minnesota Press. 1981
421. ***Andersen HK.*** Reductionism in the Biomedical Sciences. in: ***M. Solomon, JR Simon, & H Kincaid*** (eds.) The Routledge Companion to the Philosophy of Medicine. Routledge. 2017
422. ***Cartwright N.*** Against the completability of science, in: ***W.F. Stone and J Wolff*** (eds.) The Proper Ambition of Science. Routledge. 2000, pp 207–208
423. ***Hare RM***. Essay in ethical theory. Supervenience Oxford, Clarendon Press. 1989, pp 66–81. ***Shaffner K.*** Discovery and Explanation in Biology and Medicine. University of Chicago Press. 1993, pp. 461–463
424. ***D'Amico R.*** Disease and the concept of supervenience. How to understand the social construct of disease, in: ***H. Kincaid, McKitrick J.*** (eds.) Establishing Medical Reality. Springer 2007, pp. 35–45
425. ***Schaffner KF.*** The Watson-Crick model and reductionism. *British Journal of the Philosophy of Science,* **20:** 325–345, 1969
426. ***Rheinberger HJ, Müller-Wille S.*** Gene Concepts, in: ***S. Sarkar & A. Plutynski*** (eds.), A Companion to the Philosophy of Biology. Blackwell. 2008, pp. 3–21
427. ***Hull DE.*** Philosophy of biological science. Prentice Hall, 1974, p.39
428. ***Rosenberg A.*** The Structure of Biological Science. Cambridge University Press. 1985, pp. 111–117
429. ***Wittgenstein L.*** Zettel. Oxford. Basil Blackwell. 1967, §445
430. ***Wittgenstein L.*** *Tractatus logico-philosophicus.* Routledge & Kegan Paul. 1922 §6.31–6.321; 6.36f; 6.362–6.372
431. ***Wittgenstein L.*** The Blue and Brown Book. Blackwell. 1968, 23; 56–57. ***Wittgenstein L.*** Wittgenstein's Lectures. Cambridge 1932–1935. Blackwell. 1982, pp. 16; 39–40 ;70–71. ***Wittgenstein L.*** Remarks on the philosophy of psychology. Vol I Blackwell. 1980, §225. ***Wittgenstein L.*** On Certainty. Blackwell. 1969, §§12–16
432. ***Wittgenstein L.*** The Big Typescript. Blackwell, 2005, p. 417
433. ***Wittgenstein L.*** Wittgenstein's Lectures. Cambridge 1932–1935. Blackwell. 1982, p.16
434. ***Rhees R.*** Discussions of Wittgenstein. Routledge and Kegan Paul. 1970, p. 43
435. ***Wittgenstein L.*** Philosophical Investigations. Blackwell. 1968, §§43, 142
436. ***Wittgenstein L.*** Zettel. Oxford. Basil Blackwell. 1967, §438
437. ***Fine A.*** The natural ontological attitude, in ***J. Leplin*** (ed.) Scientific Realism. University of California Press.1984, pp. 83–107
438. ***Cartwright N.*** Nature, the Artful Modeler. Open Court. Chicago. 2019
439. ***Kendell RE, Jablensky A.*** Distinguishing between the validity and utility of psychiatric diagnoses. *American Journal of* ***Psychiatry****.* 2003; **160:** 4–12
440. ***Sturmberg JP.*** Knowledge Translation and Health Care—Towards Understanding its True Complexity. *International Journal of Health Policy Management.* 2018; **7:** 455–458
441. ***Danto A.*** Analytical Philosophy of Knowledge. Cambridge. Cambridge University Press. 1968; pp. 232–240
442. ***Lemoine M.*** Introduction à la philosophie des sciences médicales. Paris. Hermann. 2017

443. ***Jureidini J, McHenry LB.*** The Illusion of Evidence-Based Medicine. Exposing the crisis of credibility in clinical research. Wakefield Press. 2020. ***Jureidini J, McHenry LB.*** The illusion of evidence-based medicine. *British Medical Journal.* 2022;376:o702
444. ***Changeux JP.*** L'Homme neuronal. Fayard. 1983, ch. IX
445. ***Glannon W.*** Bioethics and the Brain. Oxford University Press. 2007, p. 8
446. ***Legrenzi P, Umiltà C.*** Neuromania. Oxford University Press. 2011
447. ***Bennett MR, Hacker PMS.*** Philosophical Foundations of Neuroscience. Blackwell. 2003
448. ***Niculescu AB, RoseberryK, Levey DF.*** Precision medicine for mood disorders: objective assessment, risk, prediction, pharmacogonomics, and repurposed drugs. *Molecular Psychiatry.* 2021, 1 April 8
449. ***Graham G.*** the Disordered Mind. An Introduction to the Philosophy of Mind and Mental Illness. Routledge. 2010, 24
450. ***Karhausen L.*** Vers une neuroscience de l'âme. Éditions Vérone. 2022
451. ***Glannon W.*** Bioethics and the Brain. Oxford University Press. 2007, pp. 29–31
452. ***Gómez JM, Nunn CL, Verdú M.*** Centrality in primate–parasite networks reveal the potential for the transmission of emerging infectious diseases to humans. *PNAS* 2013 **110:** 7738–7741, 2013
453. ***Alvergne A, Jenkinson C, Faurie C.*** (eds.) Evolutionary Thinking in Medicine. Springer. 2016
454. ***Ness RM, Williams GC.*** Why We Get Sick: The New Science of Darwinian Medicine. New York. Vintage. 1994
455. ***Gert B, Culver C.*** Defining mental disorder, in: ***J. Radden*** (ed.) The Philosophy of Psychiatry : A Companion. Oxford University Press, 2004, p. 420
456. ***Bunge M.*** Medical Philosophy. Conceptual Issues in Medicine. World Scientific Publishing Co. 2014, p. 51
457. ***Broadbent A.*** Philosophy of Medicine. Oxford University Press. 2019, p.122
458. ***Méthot P-O.*** Darwin et la médecine: intérêt et limites des explications évolutionnaires en médecine, in: ***Heams T, Huneman P, Lecointre G, Zsilberstein M.*** (eds.) Les mondes darwiniens. L'évolution de l'évolution. Editions Syllepse. 2009, pp.657–684
459. ***Ray JJ, Schulman CI.*** Fever: suppress or let it ride? *Journal of Thoracic Diseases.* **7:** 633–636, 2015
460. ***Cournoyea M.*** Evolutionary Medicine, in: ***M. Solomon, J.R. Simon, & H. Kincaid***. The Routledge Companion to Philosophy of Medicine. London. Routledge, 2017, pp. 475–486
461. ***Keyfitz N.*** Biology and demography, in: ***N. Keyfitz*** (ed.) Population and Biology: Bridge Between Disciplines. Cambridge University Press. 1984, pp. 1–7
462. ***Nesse RM & Stearns SC.*** The Great Opportunity: Evolutionary Applications to Medicine and Public Health. *Evolutionary Applications,* **1 :** 28–48, 1994
463. ***Méthot PO.*** À propos de la difficulté de définir la maladie : une perspective darwinienne, in : ***E. Giroux & M. Lemoine*** (eds.) Philosophie de la médecine. Santé, maladie, pathologie. Paris. Vrin. 2012, pp.177–213
464. ***Moore GE.*** Principia Ethica, §10 ¶ 3
465. ***Fodor J, Piatelli-Palmarni M.*** What Darwin got wrong. New York. Farrar, Straus and Giroux. 2010
466. ***Hafer A.*** The Not-So-Intelligent Designer. Eugene. Oregon. Cascade Books. 2015 p.16
467. ***Godfrey-Smith P, Wilkins JF.*** Adaptationism, in: ***S. Sarkar & A. Plutynski*** (eds.), A Companion to the Philosophy of Biology. Blackwell. 2008, pp. 186–201
468. ***Stearns SC.*** (ed.). Evolution in Health and Disease. Oxford. Oxford University Press. 1999
469. ***Nesse R.*** A propos de la difficulté de définir la maladie : une perspective darwinienne, in : ***E. Giroux & M. Lemoine.,*** (eds.) Philosophie de la médecine. Vrin. 2012, pp. 183–219
470. ***Tallis R.*** Aping Mankind. Durham. Acumen. 2011, p. 5
471. ***Midgley M.*** Evolution as a Religion. Methuen. 1985. ***Stove D.*** Darwinian Fairytales. Encounter Books. 1995. ***Dupré J.*** Darwin's Legacy. Oxford University Press. 2003. ***Charlesworth B & D.*** Evolution. Oxford University Press. 2003

472. ***Darwin C.*** On the Origin of Species by Means of Natural Selection. London. John Murray. 1859. Harvard University Press. p. 6
473. ***Tallis R.*** Aping Mankind. Durham. Acumen. 2011, p.153
474. ***Walsh DM, Lewens T, Ariew A.*** The trials of life: Natural selection and random drift. *Philosophy of Science.* **69:** 452–473, 2002
475. ***Gould SJ. & Lewontin RC.*** The spandrels of San Marco and the panglossian paradigm: a critique of the adaptationist programme. *Proceedings of the Royal Society of London.* 1979; **205**: 581–598. ***Gould SJ.*** The exaptive excellence of spandrels as a term and prototype. *Proceedings of the National Academy of Sciences.* 1991; **94:** 10750–10755
476. ***Darwin C.*** On the Origin of Species by Means of Natural Selection. London. John Murray. 1859. Harvard University Press. P.197
477. ***Hamblin CL.*** Fallacies. Methuen. 1970
478. ***Lewontin RC.*** Adaptation. Conceptual Issues in Evolutionary Biology. MIT Press, 1984
479. ***Sterelny K, Griffith PE.*** Sex and Death. An Introduction to the Philosophy of Biology. University of Chicago Press. 1999, p.22f
480. ***Schaffner KF.*** Discovery and explanation in biology and medicine. University of Chicago Press. 1993
481. ***Wittgenstein L.*** Remarques sur le Rameau d'Or de Frazer. L'Age de l'Homme. 1982, p. 21
482. ***Wittgenstein L.*** Vermischte Bemerkungen. Blackwell. 1978
483. ***Di Cesare S.*** Le naturalisme non-darwinien de Wittgenstein. 2011
484. ***Wittgenstein L.*** On Certainty. Blackwell. 1969, §253
485. ***Thoreau H.D.*** Walden, or Life in the Woods, Chapter xviii, § 14
486. ***Lemoine M.*** Introduction à la philosophie des sciences médicales. Paris. Hermann. 2017, 6
487. ***Gifford F.*** (ed.) Philosophy of Medicine. Elsevier. 2011, p.2
488. ***Simon J.*** Medical Ontology: Approaches to the Metaphysics of Medicine Dissertation, New York University (2006)2011
489. ***Stegenga J.*** Care ad Cure. University of Chicago Press. 2018b, 21
490. ***Corbellini G.*** Storia e teorie della salute e della malattia. Roma. Carocci editore. 2014
491. ***Schwarz P.*** Decision and Discovery in Defining 'Disease', p. 47–63, in: ***H. Kincaid and J. McKitrick*** (eds.) Establishing Medical Reality. Amsterdam. Springer. 2007
492. ***Cassell EJ.*** The Nature of Clinical Medicine. The Return of the Clinician. Oxford University Press. 2015
493. ***Stewart M., Brown JB., Weston WW. et al.*** Patient-Centered Medicine. Transforming the Clinical Method. Thousand Oaks, California. Sage Publications. 1995; 33
494. ***Feldman MD and Ford CV.*** Patient or Pretender. Inside the Strange World of Factitious Disorders. New York. John Wiley & Sons. 1994 Feldman MD. and Ford CV. 1994
495. ***Cassell EJ.*** The Nature of Suffering and the Goals of medicine. Oxford. Oxford University Press. 2004, p. 9
496. ***Hofmann B.*** Suffering: Harm to Bodies, Minds, and Persons, p. 129–145, in: ***T Schramme & S Edwards,*** (eds.) Volume 1, Dordrecht, Springer. 2017, 130–134
497. ***Lemoine.,*** (eds.) Philosophie de la médecine. Vrin. 2012, p.173
498. ***Broadbent A.*** Philosophy of Medicine. Oxford University Press. 2019, 183–192
499. ***Wittgenstein L.*** Philosophical Investigations. Blackwell. 1968, §243
500. ***Wittgenstein L.*** Philosophical Investigations. Blackwell. 1968, §244
501. ***Wittgenstein L.*** Philosophical Investigations. Blackwell. 1968, §256
502. ***Malcolm N.*** Knowledge of other minds. *Journal of Philosophy,* **55 :** 969–979, 1958
503. ***Wittgenstein L.*** Philosophical Investigations. Blackwell. 1968, §384
504. ***Wittgenstein L.*** Philosophical Investigations. Blackwell. 1968, §§245, 256–257
505. ***Aristotle.*** Rhetoric. Clarendon Press. 1970. 28138a 6–9
506. ***Wittgenstein L.*** Philosophical Investigations. Blackwell. 1968, §§295, 302
507. ***Hofmann B.*** Suffering: harm to bodies, Minds, and Persons, in: ***T Schramme & S Edwards.*** Handbook of the Philosophy of Medicine. Volume 1. Dordrecht. Springer. 2017, pp. 129–145

508. ***Feder KF***. in: ***M. Solomon, JR Simon, & H Kincaid*** (eds.) The Routledge Companion to the Philosophy of Medicine. Routledge. 2017, p. 432
509. ***Cassell EJ.*** The Nature of Suffering and the Goals of medicine. Oxford. Oxford University Press. 2004, p. 9
510. ***Reznek L.*** The Nature of Disease. London. Routledge. 1987, pp. 163–164
511. ***Aristote*** Metaphysics
512. ***Saint Thomas***. Livre I, Leçon XIII, in: ***J. Oesterle,*** Aristotle: On Interpretation. Commentary by St. Thomas and Cajetan, Milwaukee: Marquette University Press. 1962
513. ***Jespersen, O***. 1917. Negation in English and other languages. Copenhagen, Denmark: Høst. 1917, p.4
514. ***Ayer, AJ.*** "Negation", *Journal of Philosophy*, 49: 797–815, 1952, p.39
515. ***Strawson, PF.*** Introduction to Logical Theory, London: Methuen. 1952, p.7
516. ***Wittgenstein L.*** On Certainty. Blackwell. 1969, §27
517. ***Wittgenstein L.*** Philosophical Investigations. Blackwell. 1968, §§141, 142
518. ***Thompson RP, Upshur EG.*** Philosophy of Medicine. An Introduction. Routledge. 2018, pp. 17–23
519. ***Whelton PS, McEvoy JW, Shaw L et al.*** Association of Normal Systolic Blood Pressure Level with Cardiovascular Disease in the Absence of Risk Factors. *JAMA Cardiology.* 2020: **5**: 1011–1018
520. ***Rahimi K.*** The new data from the Blood Pressure Lowering Treatment Trialists Collaboration (BPLTTC). *European Society of Cardiology (ESC) Congress* 2020
521. ***Itoga NK, Tawfix DS, Montez-Rath ME, Chang TI.*** Contributions of Systolic and Diastolic Blood Pressure to Cardiovascular Outcomes in the ALLHAT Study. *Journal of the American College of Cardiology.* **78:** 1671–1678, 2021
522. ***Chadwick R.*** Normality as Convention and Scientific Fact, in: ***Schramme T & S Edwards S***. Handbook of the Philosophy of Medicine. Springer. 2017, pp. 17–28
523. ***Canguilhem G.*** Le normal et le pathologique. Presses universitaires de France, 1966
524. ***Rose G and Barker DJP.*** What is a case? Dichotomy or continuum? *British Medical Journal.* 1978; **2**: 873–874
525. ***Wittgenstein L.*** Philosophical Investigations. Blackwell. 1968, §122
526. ***Goosens WK.*** Values, health and medicine. *Philosophy of Science.* 1980; **47**; 100–115
527. ***Wittgenstein L.*** Notebooks 1914–1916. Blackwell. 1979, 2.8.16
528. ***Messerli FH, Shalaeva EV, Rexhaj E.*** Optimal BP Targets to Prevent Stroke and MI. Is There a Lesser of 2 Evils? *Journal of the American College of Cardiology.* **78:** 1679–1680, 2021
529. ***Plato***. The Republic of Plato, ***FM Cornford*** (ed.). Oxford. Oxford University Press. 1945, 309
530. ***Reznek L.*** The Nature of Disease. London. Routledge. 1987, 154–171. ***Boorse C.*** Health as a theoretical concept. *Philosophy of Science.* 1977 **44**: 542–573
531. ***Tranøy KE.*** Asymmetries in Ethics. *Inquiry.* 1967; **10**: 351–372
532. ***Culver CM and Gert B***. Philosophy in Medicine. Conceptual and Ethical Issues in Medicine and Psychiatry. Oxford. Oxford University Press. 1982, 27, 64–85
533. ***Austin JL.***, *Écrits philosophiques*, Seuil. 1994. p. 141
534. ***Hall TS.*** Ideas of Life and Matter. The University of Chicago Press. 19
535. ***Toulmin S.*** Foresight and Understanding. An Inquiry into the Aims of Science. London. Hutchinson of London. 1961, 56; 79
536. ***Vickers G.*** What sets the goals of public health? *The New England Journal of Medicine.* 1958; **258**: 589–596
537. ***Wittgenstein L.*** On Certainty. Blackwell. 1969
538. ***Schulte J.*** Within a System, in: ***Moyal-Sharrock D. & Brenner WH,*** (eds.) Readings of Wittgenstein *On Certainty.* Palgrave MacMillan. 2007, pp.59–75
539. ***Wittgenstein L.*** On certainty. Blackwell. 1969
540. ***Wittgenstein L.*** On certainty. Blackwell. 1969
541. ***Wittgenstein L.*** On certainty. Blackwell. 1969
542. ***Wittgenstein L.*** On certainty. Blackwell. 1969

543. ***Murray S and James MA.*** What is Hypertension? *Lancet.* **354**: pp. 593–594. 1999
544. ***Field LA.*** Mortality from Stroke and Ischemic Heart Disease Increases Exponentially with Blood Pressure. *Hypertension.* **43:** e28, 2004
545. ***Whelton PK, Carey RM et al.*** Guidelines for the Prevention, Detection, Evaluation, and Management of High Blood Pressure in Adults: A Report of the American College of Cardiology/American Association Task Force on Clinical Practice Guidelines. *Journal of the American College of Cardiology.* 2018; **71:** e127–e248
546. ***Zembic A.*** A new definition for Metabolic Healthy Obesity and risk for cardiovascular and general mortality. *JAMA Open Netw.* May 7, 2021
547. ***Wittgenstein L.*** On certainty. Blackwell. 1969
548. ***Wittgenstein L.*** *Tractatus logico-philosophicus.* Routledge & Kegan Paul. 1922. §6.13–6.421
549. ***Wittgenstein L.*** Notebooks 1914–1916. Blackwell. 1979, 24.7.16
550. ***Wittgenstein L.*** *Tractatus logico-philosophicus.* Routledge & Kegan Paul. 1922. §6.41–6.43
551. ***von Wright GH.*** The Varieties of Goodness. London. Routledge and Kegan Paul. 1963a, 56
552. ***Wittgenstein L.*** The Blue and Brown Book. Blackwell. 1968
553. ***Wittgenstein L.*** Philosophical Grammar. Blackwell. 1974, 68
554. ***Wittgenstein L.*** Philosophical Investigations. Blackwell. 1968, §§207–208; 222; 232
555. ***Boorse C.*** Wright on function. *Philosophical Review.* 1976 **85**: 70–86
556. ***Boorse C.*** Health as a theoretical concept. *Philosophy of Science.* 1977 **44**: 542–573
557. ***Hobbes T***, Leviathan or the Matter, Form & Power of a Commonwealth Ecclesiastic and Civil. 1904, I, Ch. 1, 2
558. ***Aristotle.*** Rhetoric. Clarendon Press. 1970, II, 194[a]
559. ***Wright L.*** Functions. *Philosophical Review.* **82 :** 139–168, 1973
560. ***Lemoine M.*** Introduction à la philosophie des sciences médicales. Herrmann, 2017, p.128
561. ***Spinoza B.*** Ethics, part ONE
562. ***Kant I.*** Premium Collection: Complete Critiques, Philosophical Works and Essays. 2015, 35.2.1
563. ***Kant I.*** Critique of Teleological Judgment, Oxford. Clarendon Press. 1952 II, §14
564. ***Kant I.*** Critique of Judgement. Oxford University Press. 1928, p.411
565. ***Grene M.*** The Understanding of Nature. Dordrecht. D. Reidel Publishing Company. 1974, 211
566. ***Searle JR.*** Making the Social World: The Structure of Human Civilization. Oxford University Press. 2010; 58–59
567. ***Collingwood RG***. An Essay on Metaphysics. Oxford. Clarendon Press.1940. 1998; 335–337
568. ***Margolis J.*** Negativities. The Limits of Life. Colombus. Ohio. Charles E. Merrill Publishing Company. 1975; 104
569. ***Searle JR***. The Rediscovery of Mind. London. The MIT Press. 1992; 237–239
570. ***Cartwright N.*** Nature's Capacities and their Measurement. Oxford. Oxford University Press. 1989, p. 190
571. ***McCawley JD.*** Everything that Linguists have always Wanted to Know about Logic but were afraid to ask. Oxford. Blackwell.1981, pp. 182–183
572. ***Boorse C.*** Health as a theoretical concept. *Philosophy of Science.* 1977 **44**: 542–573
573. ***Schwartz P. Schwarz P.*** Decision and Discovery in Defining 'Disease', p. 47–63, in: ***H. Kincaid and J. McKitrick*** (eds.) Establishing Medical Reality. Amsterdam. Springer. 2007. ***Boorse C.*** *Medicine and Philosophy: A Forum for Bioethics and Philosophy of Medicine*, 2017; **42**, 485–502
574. ***Smart B.*** Concepts and Causes in the Philosophy of Disease. London. Palgrave Macmillan. 2016; 39
575. ***Nordenfelt L.*** The opposition between naturalistic and holistic theories of health and disease, in: **H. Carel and R. Cooper** (eds.), Health, Illness and Disease. Philosophical Essays. London. Routledge. 2013, 24
576. ***Reznek L.*** The Nature of Disease. London. Routledge
577. ***Scheffler, I.*** The Anatomy of Inquiry. Indianapolis. Bobbs-Merrill Company. 1963, 114–115

578. ***Ruse M.*** Is Biology Different from Physics, in: ***RG Colodny*** (ed.). Logic, Laws, & Life. Some Philosophical Complications. Pittsburgh. University of Pittsburgh Press. 1977, 118–121
579. ***Schwarz P.*** Defining dysfunction: Natural selection, design, and drawing a line. *Philosophe of Science.* 2007; **74:** 364–385
580. ***Rothschild BM, Tanke D,*** **Carpenter.** Tyrannosaurs suffered from gout. 1997; *Nature*: **387**: 357
581. ***Searle JR.*** Speech Acts. Cambridge. Cambridge University Press. 1969
582. ***Monk R.*** Ludwig Wittgenstein. The Duty of a Genius. Jonathan Cape. 1990, pp. 445–450
583. ***Drury M.*** Some Notes on Conversations with Wittgenstein., in: Recollections of Wittgenstein. Oxford University Press. 1984, p. 136
584. ***Drury M.*** Some Notes on Conversations with Wittgenstein., in: Recollections of Wittgenstein. Oxford University Press. 1984, p. 154. ***Rhees R.*** Editorial Notes, in: Recollections of Wittgenstein. Oxford University Press. 1984, p. 223
585. ***Brandon RB.*** Between Saying and Doing. Towards and Analytic Pragmatism. Oxford. Oxford University Press. 2008
586. ***Cochrane AL.*** Effectiveness and Efficiency. Random Reflections on Health Services. Nuffield Trust.1972
587. ***Chapman RH, Benner JS, Petrilla AA, et al.*** Predictors of adherence with antihypertensive and lipid-lowering therapy. *Archives of Internal Medicine.* 2005 **163:** 1147–1152
588. ***Solomon M, Simon JR, Kincaid H.*** The Routledge Companion to Philosophy of Medicine. London. Routledge, 2017. ***Gifford F.*** (ed.) Philosophy of Medicine. Elsevier. 2011
589. ***Lemoine M.*** Introduction à la philosophie des sciences médicales. Herrmann, 2017
590. ***Fagot-Largeault A.*** Médecine et philosophie. Presses Universitaires de France. 2010
591. ***Cartwright N.*** What is Wrong with Bayes Nets? *The Monist.* **84:** 242)264n 2002
592. ***Hursthouse R.*** Beginning Lives. Basil Blackwell. 1987
593. ***Glover J.*** Causing Death and Saving Lifes. Penguin Books. 1977
594. ***Kohl M.*** The Morality of Killing. Humanities Press. 1974
595. ***Stegenga J.*** Medical Nihilism. Oxford University Press. 2018, p55
596. ***Dixon B.*** Beyond the Magic Bullet. London. George Allen & Unwin. 1978
597. ***Shapiro AK, Shapiro E.*** The Powerful Placebo. Baltimore. The Johns Hopkins University Press. 1997, 12
598. ***Wittgenstein L.*** Philosophical Investigations. Blackwell. 1968, §454
599. ***Hahn RA.*** The nocebo phenomenon: scope and foundations, 56–76, in : ***Harrington H*** (ed.). The Placebo Effect. Cambridge, Mass. Harvard University Press. 1997, 56–76
600. ***Gupta A, Thompson D, Whitehouse A et al.*** Adverse events associated with unblinded, but not with blinded, statin therapy in the Anglo-Scandinavian Cardiac Out comes Trial. *The Lancet.* 2017; **389 :** 2473–2481
601. ***Wittgenstein L.*** Philosophical Occasions 1912–1951, Cause and Effect. Hackett Publishing Company. 1993, p. 403
602. ***Finnis DG, Kaptchuk TJ, Miller F & Benedetti F.*** Biological, clinical and ethical advances of placebo effects. *Lancet.* 2010; **375** : 686–694
603. ***Harrington A.*** (ed.) The Placebo Effect. An Interdisciplinary Exploration. Cambridge. Harvard University Press. 1999
604. ***Ross M and Olson JM.*** An expectancy attribution model of the effects of placebos. *Psychological Review.* 1981 ; 88 : 408–437
605. ***Benedetti F, Carlino E., Pollo A.*** How Placebos change the Patient's Brain. *Neuropsychopharmacology.* 2011; **36:** 339–354
606. ***Horwitz RI, Viscoli CM, Berkman L et al.*** Treatment adherence and risk of death after myocardial infarction. *Lancet.* 1990; **336**: 542–545 Hogarthy GE et al., 1973
607. ***Coronary Drug Project Research Group.*** Influence of adherence treatment and response of cholesterol on mortality in the Coronary Drug Project. *New England Journal of Medicine.* 1980 **303:** 1038–1041

608. ***Pizzo PA, Robichaud KJ, Edwards BK, Schumaker C, Kramer BS and Johnson A.*** Oral antibiotic prophylaxis in patients with cancer: a double-blind randomized placebo-controlled trial. *Journal of Pediatrics*. 1983; **102**: 125–133
609. ***Hogarthy GE & Goldberg GE.*** Drug and sociotherapy in the aftercare of schizophrenic patients. *Archives of General Psychiatry*. 1973; **28** : 54–64
610. ***Cleophas TJM.*** The importance of placebo effects. *JAMA*. 1995 **273:** 283–284
611. ***Kirsch I.*** Specifying nonspecific psychological mechanisms of placebo effects, 166–186, in: ***Harrington, H*** (ed.) The Placebo Effect. Cambridge, Mass. Harvard University Press. 1997, 167
612. ***Frank JD.*** Persuasion and Healing. New York. Schocken Books. 1974, 136
613. **Stoessl A and de la Fuente-Fernandez R.** Willing oneself on placebo– effective on its own right. *Lancet.* 2004; **364**: 227–228
614. ***Benedetti F.*** Placebo Effects: Understanding the Mechanisms in Health and Disease. Oxford University Press. 2009
615. ***Ader***, in: ***Harrington A.*** (ed.) The Placebo Effect. An Interdisciplinary Exploration. Cambridge. Harvard University Press. 1997, 138–165
616. ***Joplin DA.*** Placebos Effects in Psychiatry and Psychotherapy. 1202–1226, in: ***KW Fulford, M Davies, RGT Gipps, et al.*** (eds.). The Oxford Handbook of Philosophy of Psychiatry. 2013, 1218–1219
617. ***Lamee R, Thompson D, Dheby H-M, et al.*** Percutaneous coronary intervention instable angina (ORBITA) : a double-blind, randomized controlled trial. *Lancet.* 2018 ; **391 :** 31–40
618. ***Wittgenstein L.*** Vermischte Bemerkungen. Blackwell. 1978
619. ***Maughan S.*** Human Bondage, Ch LIV
620. ***Shaffer MJ.*** Counterfactuals and Scientific Realism. Palgrave. Macmillan. 2012
621. ***Lewis D.*** Causation. *Journal of Philosophy.* **70:** 556–567, 1973
622. ***Toulmin S, Rieke R and Janik A.*** An introduction to reasoning. New York. Macmillan Publishing Co 1979, p.235
623. ***Toulmin S.*** Foresight and Understanding. An Inquiry into the Aims of Science. London. Hutchinson of London. 1961, 43
624. ***Toulmin S, Rieke R and Janik A.*** An introduction to reasoning. New York. Macmillan Publishing Co. 1979, p.79
625. ***Toulmin S, Rieke R and Janik A.*** An introduction to reasoning. New York. Macmillan Publishing Co. 1979, p.63
626. ***Wittgenstein L.*** The Blue and Brown Book. Blackwell. 1968
627. ***Wittgenstein L.*** The Blue and Brown Book. Blackwell. 1968
628. ***Wittgenstein L.*** Philosophical Investigations. Blackwell. 1968, §65
629. ***Wittgenstein L.*** Philosophical Investigations. Blackwell. 1968, §52
630. ***Wittgenstein L.*** Philosophical Investigations. Blackwell. 1968, §66
631. ***Wittgenstein L.*** The Blue and Brown Book. Blackwell. 1968
632. ***Wittgenstein L.*** The Blue and Brown Book. Blackwell. 1968
633. ***Wittgenstein L.*** On certainty. Blackwell. 1969, §61
634. ***Wittgenstein L.*** Remarks on the Foundations of Mathematics. Blackwell, 1967, §134, p. 90
635. ***Wittgenstein L.*** Philosophical Investigations. Blackwell. 1968, §71
636. ***Wittgenstein L.*** The Blue and Brown Book. Blackwell. 1968
637. ***Wittgenstein L.*** Philosophical Investigations. Blackwell. 1968, §§ 70–91
638. ***Wittgenstein L.*** Philosophical Investigations. Blackwell. 1968, §71
639. ***Hacking I.*** Tradition of Natural Kinds. *Philosopical Studies.* Vol lxi. 1991
640. ***Ereshefsky M.*** Systematics and Taxonomy, in: ***S. Sarkar & A. Plutynski*** (eds.), A Companion to the Philosophy of Biology. Blackwell. 2008, pp. 99–107
641. ***Dupré J.*** Natural Kinds and Biological Taxa, in: The Disorder of Things. Harvard University Press. 1995
642. ***Wittgenstein L.*** The Blue and Brown Book. Blackwell. 1968
643. ***Wittgenstein L.*** Philosophical Remarks. Blackwell. 1975, p. 269

644. ***Aucouturier V, Demazeux S.*** The Concept of "Mental Disorder", in: ***H. Carel, Cooper R.*** (eds.) Health, Illness and Disease. Routledge. 2013, p. 78
645. ***Wittgenstein L.*** Philosophical Investigations. Blackwell. 1968, p. 294
646. ***Rosch E. and Mervis CB.*** Family Resemblances. Studies in the Internal Structure of Categories. *Cognitive Psychology,* **7 :** 573–605, 1975
647. ***Wittgenstein L.*** Philosophical Investigations. Blackwell. 1968, §§73, 74
648. ***Sadegh-Zadeh K.*** La théorie de la maladie comme ressemblance à un prototype in : ***E. Giroux & M. Lemoine.,*** (eds.) Philosophie de la médecine. Vrin. 2012, pp. 369–404
649. ***Black M.*** Language and Philosophy. Cornell University Press. 1949, pp. 23–58
650. ***Zadeh L.*** Logic and Approximate Reasoning. *Synthese* **90 :** 409–410, 1975
651. ***Sadegh-Zadeh K.*** La théorie de la maladie comme ressemblance à un prototype in : ***E. Giroux & M. Lemoine.,*** (eds.) Philosophie de la médecine. Vrin. 2012, pp. 369–404
652. ***Wittgenstein L.*** Philosophical Grammar. Blackwell. 1974, §70
653. ***Wittgenstein L.*** Philosophical Investigations. Blackwell. 1968, §135
654. ***Aristotle.*** The Physics. Harvard University Press. 1957, 209a15ff
655. ***Lakoff G.*** Women, Fire and Dangerous Things: What Categories Reveal about the Mind/ University of Chicago Press. 1987, p. 6
656. ***Klagge JC.*** Wittgenstein in Exile. The MIT Press. 2011, p. 213, n.6
657. ***Wittgenstein L.*** Philosophical Remarks. Blackwell. 1975, p. 263
658. ***Hofman B.*** Do health professionals have a prototype concept of disease? The answer is no. *Philosophy, Ethics, and Humanities in Medicine.* **12:** 1, article 6, 2017
659. ***Lilienfeld SO, Marino L.*** Mental Disorder as a Roschian Concept: a Critique of Wakefield's "Harmful Dysfunction" Analysis. *Journal of Abnormal Psychology.* **104:** 411–420, 1995
660. ***Thompson P.*** Theories and Models in Medicine, in: ***Gifford F.*** (ed.) Philosophy of Medicine. Elsevier. 2011, pp. 116–136
661. ***Van Fraasen B.*** The Scientific Image. Oxford University Press. 1980
662. ***Cartwright N.*** Nature, the Artful Modeler. Open Court. Chicago. 2019
663. ***Karhausen L.*** Dr Georges Canguilhem Médecin anomal. Paris. L'Harmattan, 1997, pp. 172–177
664. ***Bunge M.*** Medical Philosophy. Conceptual Issues in Medicine. World Scientific Publishing Co. 2014, pp. 58–59
665. ***Canguilhem G.*** Le normal et le pathologique. Presses universitaires de France, 1966, p. 91. ***Canguilhem G.*** Études d'histoire et de philosophie des sciences. Paris. Vrin. 2015
666. ***Karhausen L.*** Dr Georges Canguilhem Médecin anomal. Paris. L'Harmattan, 1997, pp. 136–139
667. ***Gaille M.*** Philosophie de la médecine. Vol. 1. Frontières, savoir, clinique. VRIN. 2011. ***Giroux E, Lemoine M.*** Philosophie de la médecine. Vol. 2. Santé, maladie, pathologie. VRIN. 2012
668. ***Hippocrate.*** Les œuvres d'Hippocrate. Traduites en François. Tome premier. Paris. Par la Compagnie des Libraires. 1697

MIX
Papier aus verantwortungsvollen Quellen
Paper from responsible sources
FSC® C105338

If you have any concerns about our products,
you can contact us on
ProductSafety@springernature.com

In case Publisher is established outside the EU,
the EU authorized representative is:
Springer Nature Customer Service Center GmbH
Europaplatz 3, 69115 Heidelberg, Germany

Printed by Libri Plureos GmbH
in Hamburg, Germany